Tumors of Skin
Appendages

Practical Dermatopathology Series

Lymphoproliferative Disorders of the Skin
edited by George F. Murphy and Martin C. Mihm, Jr.

Tumors of Skin Appendages
by Ken Hashimoto, Amir H. Mehregan, and Masanobu Kumakiri

Pediatric Dermatopathology
by George F. Murphy and Martin C. Mihm, Jr.

Tumors of Skin Appendages

KEN HASHIMOTO, M.D.

Professor and Chairman, Department of Dermatology and Syphilology, Wayne State University School of Medicine, Detroit, Michigan

AMIR H. MEHREGAN, M.D.

Clinical Professor of Dermatology and Syphilology, Wayne State University School of Medicine, Detroit, Michigan

MASANOBU KUMAKIRI, M.D.

Associate Professor of Dermatology, Hokkaido University School of Medicine, Sapporo, Japan

Butterworths

Boston   London   Durban   Singapore   Sydney   Toronto   Wellington

Every effort has been made to ensure that the drug
dosage schedules within this text are accurate and
conform to standards accepted at time of publication.
However, as treatment recommendations vary in the
light of continuing research and clinical experience,
the reader is advised to verify drug dosage schedules
herein with information found on product information
sheets. This is especially true in cases of new or
infrequently used drugs.

Library of Congress Cataloging-in-Publication Data

Hashimoto, Ken, 1931–
  Tumors of skin appendages.

  (Practical dermatopathology series)
  Includes bibliographies and index.
  1. Exocrine glands—Tumors. 2. Skin—Tumors.
3. Hair follicles—Tumors. I. Mehregan, Amir H.
II. Kumakiri, Masanobu. III. Title. IV. Series:
Practical dermatopathology series. [DNLM: 1. Skin
Neoplasms. WR 500 H348t]
RC280.S5H32 1987   616.99'277   86–26877
ISBN 0–409–95159–5

Butterworth Publishers
80 Montvale Avenue
Stoneham, MA 02180

10 9 8 7 6 5 4 3 2 1

Printed in the United States of America

This work is dedicated to Walter F. Lever, M.D., and the late Hermann Pinkus, M.D.

Contents

Preface

Many changes have taken place since *Appendage Tumors of the Skin* by Ken Hashimoto and Walter F. Lever was published in 1968. New entities have been discovered, new methodologies applied, and the histogenesis of some tumors has been clarified. No doubt, the next five to ten years will see a vast expansion of this research area through DNA hybridization, oncogene cloning, and applications of still undeveloped methodologies. No previous decade of medical research has produced so much high-quality information as the past ten years. We are in the most exciting and, in a way, most fluctuating era of medical science. On the other hand, morphological description remains the basis of pathology and, despite ever-changing interpretation, has permanent value. Many pictures published in the first edition of Lever's textbook have continued to appear in subsequent editions; under new interpretations, old pictures appear as fresh as brand new photographs.

The purpose of this book is to capture today's concepts in this old discipline and simultaneously to gather and interpret information for many conflicting, redundant entities. In so doing, we were bound to be subjective (and even a bit dogmatic), critical and selective, although we tried hard to make this volume a consensus opinion of the 1980s.

The materials used are largely derived from our collections but many came from friends. Without their help, this work would never have been completed.

The photography done by Dr. Soo Duk Lee and Mr. David Snaddon and the typing performed by Mrs. Eleanor Chiesa are also acknowledged. This work is supported in part by a Veterans Administration Merit Review Research Grant.

K. H.

1

Histogenesis of Adnexal Tumors

The appendage tumors are a group of skin tumors whose structures resemble normal mature skin appendages such as hair and the sweat and sebaceous glands (Tables 1.1 and 1.2). These tumors may have emerged from the preexisting adnexal structures by dedifferentiation. Figure 1.1, showing an inverted follicular keratosis connected to a hair follicle, and Figure 1.2, demonstrating a pilomatricoma connected to a hair follicle, illustrate the development of some appendage tumors, usually well-differentiated varieties, from the preexisting structures. Figure 1.3 shows an epithelial cyst connected to an enlarged hair follicle. The upper part of the cyst shows infundibular (or epidermoid) keratinization, and the lower part is walled by isthmic epithelium, revealing trichilemmal keratinization. This type of cyst is called hybrid cyst (see page 103). The attached follicular structure resembles the outer root sheath or trichilemma. These examples clearly demonstrate that normal skin appendages and their neoplasms are closely related.

Less convincing but better than coincidental findings are the coexistence of eccrine ducts adjacent to an eccrine hidrocystoma (Fig. 2.30) and the presence of apocrine glands in the vicinity of an apocrine cystadenoma. These ducts and glands often connect with cystic lesions. Ectopic apocrine glands often underlie syringocystadenoma papilliferum, suggesting that they are interrelated.

Table 1.1
Classification of skin appendage tumors

Tumor	Eccrine differentiation	Hair differentiation	Sebaceous differentiation	Apocrine differentiation
Mature tumors Hyperplasia Hamartomas Organic Nevus	Eccrine nevus Eccrine duct proliferation Eccrine-centered nevus Eccrine angiomatous hamartoma Syringofibroadenoma or acrosyringeal nevus Comedo nevus of the palm, linear eccrine nevus with comedone, porokeratotic eccrine ostial nevus, or porokeratotic eccrine duct and hair follicle nevus	Hair follicle nevus Nevus comedonicus Fibrofolliculoma Perifollicular fibroma Arrector pili muscle hamartoma Facial milium	Nevus sebaceus Senile sebaceous hyperplasia, Fordyce's spots (granules or condition) Premature sebaceous gland hyperplasia	Apocrine nevus
Less mature tumors Adenoma Organoid	Eccrine adenoma Eccrine hidrocystoma or cystadenoma Syringoma: classic eyelid type, eruptive hidradenoma, clear cell type, chondroid type Papillary eccrine adenoma (eccrine syringocystadenoma papilliferum) (cutaneous ciliated cyst)	Trichofolliculoma Sebaceous trichofolliculoma Eruptive vellus hair cyst Trichostasis spinulosa Fibrofolliculoma Perifollicular fibroma Trichodiscoma Becker's pigmented hairy nevus or Becker's melanosis Dilated pore of Winer Pilar sheath acanthoma	Sebaceous adenoma Sebaceoma	Apocrine hidrocystoma or apocrine cystadenoma, Moll's gland cyst Hidradenoma papilliferum Tubular apocrine adenoma Erosive adenomatosis of the nipple Apocrine adenoma and ceruminous adenoma Apocrine fibroadenoma Apocrine syringocyst-adenoma papilliferum

Least mature tumors Epitheliomas Suborganoid Borderline carcinomas				
Eccrine poroma	Trichoepithelioma, desmoplastic trichoepithelioma	Sebaceous epithelioma	Dermal cylindroma
Eccrine poromatosis	Trichoadenoma	Sebaceous differentiation of basal cell epithelioma	Apocrine chondroid syringoma
Solid-cystic hidradenoma	Trichilemmal cyst, hybrid cyst, proliferating trichilemmal cyst		Apocrine differentiation of basal cell epithelioma
Hidroacanthoma simplex	Trichilemmoma		(Extramammary Paget's disease)
Syringoacanthoma	Steatocystoma multiplex		
Dermal duct tumor	Inverted follicular keratosis		
Eccrine spiradenoma	Pilomatricoma (calcifying epithelioma)		
Clear cell hidradenoma (eccrine acrospiroma)	Tumor of follicular infundibulum		
Eccrine chondroid syringoma	Keratotic basal cell epithelioma		
Aggressive digital papillary adenoma	Trichoblastoma-trichogenic trichoblastoma		
Eccrine differentiation of basal cell epithelioma (eccrine dermal cylindroma)	Trichoblastic fibroma		
	Basaloid follicular hamartoma		
	Pilomatricoma		

Table 1.2
Malignant tumors of skin appendages

Eccrine gland	Sebaceous gland	Apocrine gland
Primary eccrine adenocarcinomas Solid-cellular, adenoid-cystic, microcystic, tubular, basalioma-like, squamoid	Sebaceous carcinoma	Apocrine adenocarcinoma Malignant hidroadenoma papilliferum Extramammary Paget's disease
Syringoid eccrine carcinoma		
Clear cell eccrine carcinoma		
Mucinous eccrine carcinoma		
Malignant eccrine spiradenoma		
Porocarcinoma		
Malignant syringoacanthoma		
Malignant chondroid syringoma		
Aggressive digital adenocarcinoma		

On the other hand, some appendage tumors, particularly immature varieties, may arise from any of the adnexa; matrix cells of these structures are immature and pluripotential. They are also noncommitted and are therefore equipotential.[1,2,3] Stated differently, matrix cells of one adnexal structure can differentiate into another structure. It may not be surprising that matrix cells of an eccrine duct can renew the straight duct, acrosyringium, and epidermis,[4] or that human vellus hair follicles may regenerate from the upper portion of large hair follicles during wound healing,[5,6] because in these instances the regeneration takes place within the same appendage. More striking evidence of pluripotentiality of matrix cells was recently shown by the transformation of trichilemmoma cells into eccrine gland cells in vitro.[7]

The skin area where adnexal tumors develop seems to be a special neoplastic environment or a field of neoplasia.[7,8] Nevus sebaceus lesions are often complicated by the development of a variety of adnexal tumors and basal cell epitheliomas. Such "hot spots" in the skin may extend locally or linearly as in linear epidermal nevus or basaloid follicular hamartoma[9] (Figure 1.4). Examples of local fields of neoplasia are multiple trichoepithelioma, adenoma sebaceum (angiofibroma), or trichilemmomas of Cowden's syndrome.

As with many neoplasms, the causes of these tumors are unknown. Chemical carcinogens or viruses[10] can be the causes in susceptible individuals and families. Most spontaneous tumors seem to be of monoclonal origin, whereas many inherited tumors are polyclonal.[11] Benign tumors tend to be polyclonal and malignant ones monoclonal.[12,13] Because many benign adnexal tumors are hereditary and benign, they are most likely polyclonal; in fact, trichoepithelioma[14] and hereditary neurofibroma[15] have been reported to be polyclonal.

In the hereditary tumors the first stage of tumorigenesis is already built into the germinal cells and inherited. It has been postulated that the second stage is a mutational transformation of genetically abnormal somatic cells.[11] In benign adnexal tumors, mutational changes may occur simultaneously or

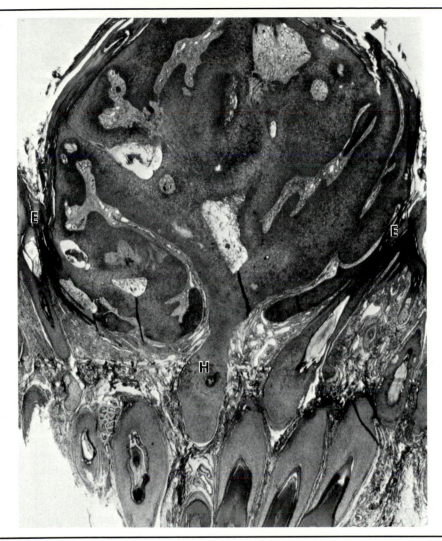

Figure 1.1
Inverted follicular keratosis. A round ball-like growth extends from the skin surface into the dermis. The growth consists of massive proliferation of follicular sheath epithelium that connects with a hair follicle (H) and surrounding epidermis (E). The connection to a hair follicle suggests that this lesion has grown out of a pre-existing structure of this follicle (× 24).

in sequence in the many matrix cells that are genetically at risk. The best example of sequential development of a second-stage abnormality would be nevus sebaceus (organoid nevus). In this case the initial lesion of hyperplastic epidermis in which pilosebaceous structures develop abnormally is followed by neoplastic development of the sebaceous gland, hair structures, the apocrine gland, and finally basal cell epithelioma. All somatic cells should contain an equal amount of genetic defects inherited from abnormal germinal cells.

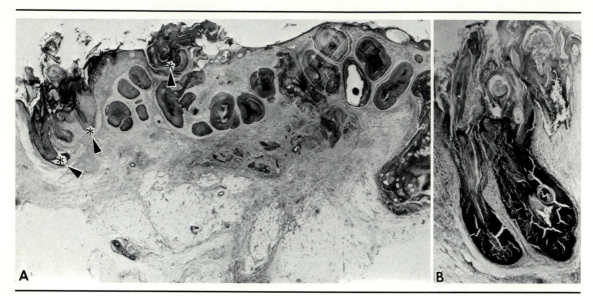

Figure 1.2
Calcifying epithelioma or pilomatricoma. Intradermal lesions are communicated to the surface where hair follicle-like structures (arrowheads and asterisks in A) are formed. Two structures shown in B could be taken as hair follicles. See Figure 3.22 for more details. (A × 6 and B × 10.) (Courtesy of Akinobu Shoji, M.D., and Toshio Hamada, M.D.)

However, location, patient age, and exposure to ultraviolet light or other noxious agents influence the expression of abnormal genes. For example, multiple trichoepitheliomas always occur on the face, eccrine poromas most frequently on the palms and soles, and steatocystoma multiplex affects the skin of the sternum, axilla, and genitalia. Obviously, the adnexa related to these tumors are more concentrated in these specific areas and the chances of abnormal genes becoming manifest are greater there than in other locations. However, the reason why the scalp, where hair and sebaceous glands abound, is not involved in multiple trichoepithelioma and steatocystoma multiplex needs explanation. It may be that defective genes for these tumors prefer small

Figure 1.3
Hybrid cyst. (A) An intradermal cyst is seen attached to the tail of a hair follicle (H) and hair papilla (P) in low magnification. The wall of this cyst undergoes epidermoid (upper part between arrowheads) or trichilemmal keratinization (the rest of the wall). In a serial section this cyst was found to open (O) to the skin surface (A inset). The two junctions (1, 2 of A) between trichilemmal and epidermoid keratinization are enlarged in B and C. Under the polarized light trichilemmal keratin exhibits a stronger birefringence (D, E). The hair follicle-like attachment in A is enlarged in F and resembles the cylindrical type of trichilemmoma (see Fig. 3.5). (A × 24; Inset, × 24; B–E, × 63; F, × 200.) (Courtesy of Homayoon Rahbari, M.D.)

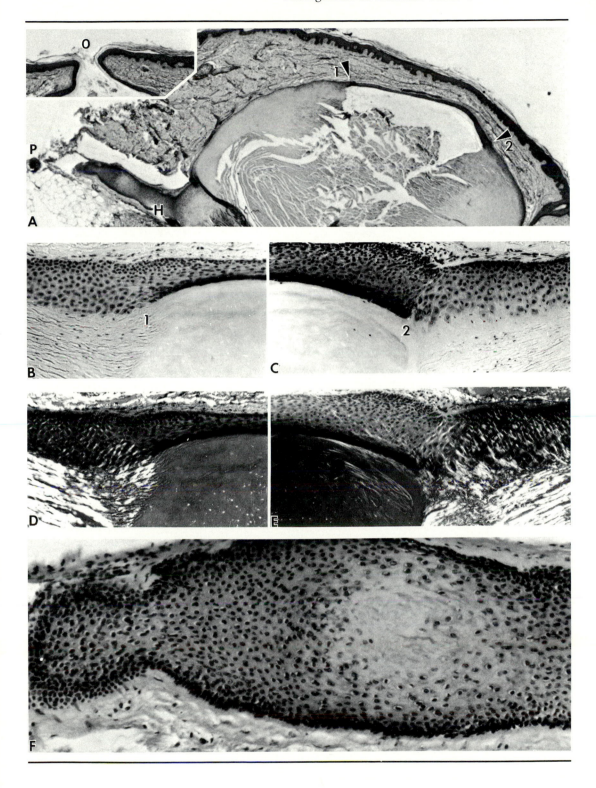

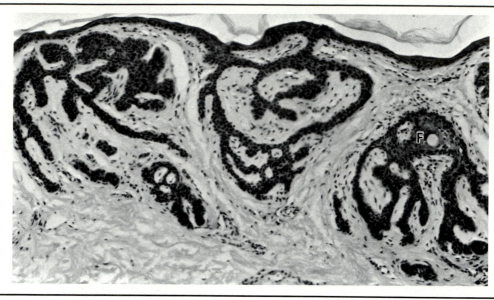

Figure 1.4
Basaloid follicular hamartoma. Each vellus hair follicle (F) in this field of neoplasia is transformed into anastomosing epithelial cords of basaloid cells. Individual follicular lesions resemble basal cell epithelioma not only in their small basophilic cells but also in their well-organized stroma. (× 30). (From Mehregan AH, Baker S. Basaloid Follicular Hamartoma. J Cutan Pathol 1985;12:55. © 1985 Munksgaard International Publishers Ltd, Copenhagen, Denmark.)

vellus to large terminal hairs for their oncogenic expression. In familial eruptive syringoma[16] only those eccrine gland cells that are located in the neck, umbilical area, genitalia, and later in the eyelids undergo second-stage transformation. Cells in the palms and soles, though equally defective genetically, are unaffected. In general, appendage tumors that occur in multiple numbers, such as trichoepithelioma, are familial, probably because the inherited abnormal genes are ubiquitous and are expressed in all their target organs, such as vellus hair follicles in the case of trichoepithelioma.

The classification of adnexal tumors is based on both the direction and degree of their differentiation (Table 1.1). The criteria for differentiation used to be based on histologic resemblance between the tumor and normal skin appendages. With the advent of histochemistry and electron microscopy, functional aspects (Table 1.3) and fine structural criteria (Table 1.4) were added to this pattern analysis,[17] and immunohistochemistry using monoclonal and polyclonal antibodies against specific components of the tumor cells has recently gained popularity[18] (Table 1.5). For example, syringoma exhibits lumen-forming epithelial islands in the upper dermis. Some lumina are connected to the epidermis and contain keratin. These histologic findings suggest but do not confirm the differentiation of syringoma toward eccrine duct in the upper dermis or acrosyringium. Ultrastructural analysis shows that the epithelial cells surrounding these lumina contain lysosomes, and that intracellular cavity

Table 1.3
Patterns of enzymatic reactions in adult eccrine and apocrine glands

Stain	Eccrine secretory segment	Eccrine duct	Apocrine secretory segment	Apocrine duct
Amylophosphorylase and branching enzyme	++++	++++	-~+	++
Succinic dehydrogenase	+++	+++	+	-
Leucine aminopeptidase	++++	+++	++	+
PAS	++++	+++	+	+++
Diastase-resistant PAS	+++ lumen++++	++ cuticle+++	some granules++ lumen++	+ cuticle+++
Acid phosphatase	++	++	++++	+++
Indoxyl esterase	+	+	++	-
Alkaline phosphatase	- myoepithelial++++ cells	-	- myoepithelial++++ cells	-
β-Glucuronidase	-	-	+++	+

No reaction: -
Weak reaction: +
Moderate reaction: ++
Strong reaction: +++
Very strong reaction: ++++

Table 1.4
Ultrastructural differentiation of the luminal cells of eccrine and apocrine glands

Site	Luminal villi	Multivesicular dense bodies (lysosomes)	Annulate lamellae	Secretory granules	Perluminal filamentous zone	Secretory cell	Myoepithelial cell
Embryo eccrine duct in lower epidermis	++++	++++			+++		–
Adult eccrine duct in lower epidermis	+++	+			++++		–
Regenerating eccrine duct in epidermis	+++	++++			+++		
Embryo eccrine duct in dermis	++	–			+		–
Embryo eccrine secretory segment	+	–			–		– + at 20 weeks
Adult eccrine secretory segment	++	–	–	1. Uniformly sized dense to light granules (mucous cell) 2. Small number of large lipid granules	–	1. Glycogen-rich clear cell (serous cell) 2. Glycogen-free dense cell (mucous cell)	+++
Embryo apocrine duct	+	+ (intrafollicular portion)			+		–
Adult apocrine duct	++	+ (intrafollicular portion)			+++		–
Embryo apocrine secretory segment	+	–	+++		–		+ at 24 weeks
Adult apocrine	++	–		1. Light mitochondrial granule 2. Dense lysosomal granules that may be gigantic in size	–	1. Tall columnar cells with small amount of glycogen; decapitation secretion of apex	

Table 1.5
Immunohistochemical methods for eccrine and apocrine glands

| Stain | Eccrine | | Apocrine | |
	Secretory	Duct	Secretory	Duct
CEA	+ + +	+ + +	+ + +	+ + +
S100	+ + +	−	−	−
EKH4	+ + + (myoepithelial cells)	+	+ + + (myoepithelial cells)	+
EKH5	+ + +	−	±	−
EKH6	+ + +	+ + + (coiled duct)	− ~ +	− ~ +
AN3	+ + + (myoepithelial cells)	−	+ + + (myoepithelial cells)	−
GCDFP-15	−	−	+ + +	+ + +

EKH4: This monoclonal antibody recognized 50 Kd keratin and thus also labels basal cells of the epidermis.

CEA: Carcinoembryonic antigen. Lumen-forming type or tubulocystic portion of most appendage tumors contain CEA. Paget's cells are positive.

S100: Positive in 40% to 50% of eccrine spiradenoma tumor cells.

GCDFP-15: Gross cystic disease fluid protein of the breast.

formation initiates the lumen formation; thus, they closely resemble the embryonic acrosyringium (Table 1.4). A histochemical panel of eccrine-type enzymes is positive in the epithelial islands, as is eccrine-specific monoclonal antibody. All available analytic methods thus support an eccrine differentiation, particularly toward the acrosyringeal portion, in syringoma. In such comparative analysis it is implicitly agreed that the transformed adnexal structures and cells share the same morphological, functional, and antigenic characteristics as are commonly found in their normal counterparts.

In well-differentiated adnexal tumors such as syringoma, trichilemmal cysts, and epidermoid cysts, the degree of resemblance to the normal structure is sufficient for diagnosis; H & E stain alone can tell their direction of differentiation. Less differentiated tumors such as eccrine spiradenoma, clear cell hidradenoma, and pilomatricoma require ultrastructural, histochemical, and/or immunohistochemical analyses. Very immature tumors such as dermal cylindroma still defy final classification because they show little specific differentiation despite the application of various investigative techniques. In eccrine spiradenoma myoepithelial cells are always present, albeit few in number. In dermal cylindroma they are absent, even under the secretory epithelium that lines the lumen. In apocrine hidrocystoma myoepithelial cells line the basal layer, whereas in Moll's gland cysts and syringocystadenoma papilliferum they are undeveloped even though some parts of their cystic or tubular walls are lined with secretory epithelium. Because myoepithelial cells of the eccrine and apocrine glands develop from the basal keratinocytes of the embryonic ducts as a primordial glandular coil is formed at the tip of the elongating duct,[19] the presence or absence of typical myoepithelial cells seems to depend upon how far these immature basal cells eventually differentiate and synthesize myosin instead of keratin. Hybrid cells containing both keratin and my-ofibrils have been found in embryonic sweat glands.[19] Myoepithlial cells may undergo an atrophic degeneration under pressure: Their absence in expanding cystic lesions without open duct may be due to this mechanism, as postulated in Moll's gland cyst (page 153).

Although the classification of adnexal tumors has been largely of academic interest, there are many occasions when a precise diagnosis of adnexal tumors is of the utmost clinical importance. An example is differentiation of seba-ceous gland carcinoma from metastatic lesions such as renal cell carcinoma. Eccrine sweat gland carcinoma has often been confused with metastatic ad-enocarcinomas or Merkel cell carcinoma. In adnexal carcinomas, many of which are highly malignant, the correct diagnosis may depend upon the de-tection and definition of preexisting benign appendage tumors that may be found in some part of the same lesion.

Based on an assumption that cells from each definable segment of the ad-nexa may give rise to tumors ranging from benign to malignant, one can construct a "periodical table of adnexal tumors."[20] In this classification, the specific segments of normal adnexa that these tumors resemble and their de-gree of differentiation (Table 1.1) have been used as basic criteria. The term "adenoma" as used in Table 1.1 may not be applicable to solid tumors such as sebaceous adenoma because adenoma means a glandular tumor of lesser maturity. However, conventional names are sometimes difficult to change and therefore used as such. This table is not as complete as the periodical table of the elements; however, if one counts rare tumors or tumor parts, the table will probably be completed in the near future. This method of classification is used in the following chapters of this monograph.

REFERENCES

1. Pinkus H. Premalignant fibroepithelial tumors of skin. Arch Derm Syph 1953; 67:598–615.
2. Pinkus H. Clinical, histological and differential considerations. In: Rothman S, ed. Human integument. Washington, D.C.: Amer Assoc Adv Science, 1959.
3. Montagna W. Structure and function of skin. New York: Academic Press, 1962.
4. Lobitz WC, Holyoke JB, Montagna W. Responses of the human eccrine sweat duct to controlled injury. J Invest Dermatol 1954;23:329–344.
5. Kligman AM, Strauss JS. The formation of vellus hair follicles from human adult epidermis. J Invest Dermatol 1956;27:19–23.
6. Inaba M, Anthony J, McKinstry C. Histologic study of the regeneration of axillary hair after removal with subcutaneous tissue shaver. J Invest Dermatol 1979;72:224.
7. Hashimoto K, Kanzaki T. Appendage tumors of the skin: histogenesis and ultra-structure. J Cutan Pathol 1984;11:365–381.
8. Mehregan AH. The origin of the adnexal tumors of the skin. A viewpoint. J Cutan Pathol 1985;12:459–467.
9. Mehregan AH, Baker S. Basaloid follicular hamartoma. Report of 3 cases with localized and systematized unilateral lesions. J Cutan Pathol 1985;12:55–65.
10. Hashimoto K, Magre LA, Lever WF. Electron microscopic identification of viral particles in calcifying epithelioma induced by polyoma virus. J Natl Cancer Inst 1967;39:977–992.

11. Hsu SH, Luk GD, Krush AJ, Hamilton SR, Hoover HH. Multiclonal origin of polyps in Gardner syndrome. Science 1983;221:951–953.
12. Friedman JM, Fialkow PJ, Greene GI, Weinberg MN. Probable clonal origin of neurofibrosarcoma in a patient with hereditary neurofibromatosis. J Natl Cancer Inst 1982;69:1289–1291.
13. Moolgavkar SH, Knudson AG. Mutation and cancer: A model for human carcinogenesis. J Natl Cancer Inst 1981;66:1037–1052.
14. Gartler SM, Ziprkowski L, Krakowski A, Ezra R, Szeinberg A, Adam A. Glucose-6-phosphate dehydrogenase mosaicism as a tracer in the study of hereditary multiple trichoepithelioma. Am J Hum Genet 1966;18:282–287.
15. Fialkow PJ, Sagebiel RW, Gartler SM, Rimoin DL. Multiple cell origin of hereditary neurofibromas. N Engl J Med 1971;284:298–300.
16. Hashimoto K, Blum D, Fukaya T, Eto H. Familial syringoma: case history and application of monoclonal anti-eccrine gland antibodies. Arch Dermatol 1985;121:756–760.
17. Hashimoto K, Lever WF. Appendage tumors of the skin. 1968; Springfield, Il: Charles C. Thomas.
18. Hashimoto K, Eto H, Matsumoto M, Hori K. Anti-keratin monoclonal antibodies: production, specificities and applications. J Cutan Pathol 1983;10:529–539.
19. Hori K, Hashimoto K, Eto H, Dekio S. Keratin type intermediate filaments in sweat gland myoepithelial cells. J Invest Dermatol 1985;85:453–549.
20. Lever WF, Schaumburg-Lever G. Histopathology of the skin. 6th ed, 1983; Philadelphia: JB Lippincott, 523.

2

Eccrine Gland Tumors

During the third to fifth months of fetal life eccrine glands develop, first on the palms and soles, then in the axillae, and finally in the rest of the body. From the undersurface of the epidermis eccrine germs emerge as offshoots of the basal cells. Just above these buds a concentric group of epidermal cells is seen; these resemble squamous eddies except that, in the inner cells, small cavities constituting the primordial intraepidermal duct are formed. These cavities are produced by lysosomal digestion of the cytoplasm. The base of the eccrine germs forms eccrine ridges, which are wider and extend more deeply into the dermis than the regular epidermal rete ridges. The eccrine ridge and the cells of the intraepidermal duct wall form a specialized unit that reproduces itself by mitosis of the basal cells of the eccrine ridge; this unit is called the *acrosyringium*. Tumors that mimic the acrosyringium are eccrine poroma, hidroacanthoma simplex, syringoacanthoma, and others. Nevoid hyperplasia of the acrosyringium is seen in several conditions such as acrosyringial nevus, porokeratotic eccrine ostial and dermal duct nevus, comedo nevus of the palm, and porokeratotic eccrine duct and hair follicle nevus, among others. Tumors that show differentiation toward the eccrine ridge and upper dermal duct include syringoma, dermal duct tumor, and some varieties of clear cell hidradenoma.

As eccrine germs elongate, they grow relatively straight down to the junction between the dermis and subcutaneous fat tissue, where the tip of each eccrine germ develops into a swollen bulb and the distal point begins to coil upon itself. The straight duct and the coiled duct are thus produced. The swollen end continues to elongate and simultaneously coil; this portion becomes the secretory segment. The ductal lumen is produced by detachment of the inner cells. The secretory segment differentiates into three cell types: clear (serous) cells, dark (mucous) cells, and myoepithelial cells. Dilatation of the straight dermal duct causes eccrine hidrocystoma or eccrine cystadenoma. Adenomatous growth of the eccrine duct, particularly of the lower portion, causes papillary eccrine adenoma. Tumors of the secretory portion may include eccrine spiradenoma, some varieties of clear cell hidradenoma, eccrine adenomas, and various types of eccrine adenocarcinoma.

Morphologic variations are so great from one variety to another that there are no uniform criteria to diagnose eccrine gland tumors. However, their tendency to form lumina, the presence of clear cells with high glycogen content, and their lesser propensity for keratinization may be helpful in differentiating eccrine gland tumors from hair follicle tumors which may contain glycogen-rich clear cells but no lumina. Histochemical and immunohistochemical stains have been very helpful (Tables 1.3, 1.5) and will increase in value as more and more new antibodies are developed. Ultrastructural observations can not only facilitate identification of the eccrine nature of some tumors but also can specify the portion of the eccrine gland toward which the tumors are differentiating (Table 1.4).

Eccrine Poroma

A major class of eccrine sweat gland tumors is the eccrine poroma group, or tumors of the acrosyringium. These are the tumors which differentiate toward the most distal segment of the eccrine sweat gland.

Eccrine poroma was first described by Pinkus et al.[1] It occurs in both sexes, usually past age 40, on palmar or plantar skin[2] where eccrine glands are abundant. Less frequently, lesions have been reported in other anatomical sites such as the neck, chest, back, calves, popliteal region, nose, and occasionally within a site of chronic radiation dermatitis.[3,4] The tumors are dome-shaped, sessile, or verrucous (Fig. 2.1) and measure less than 3 cm in diameter. Their surface is either crusted or eroded. Removal of the crust reveals an angiomatous, easily bleeding, rubbery tumor (Fig. 2.1). The growth is asymptomatic.

Histopathology

In classic eccrine poroma as originally described by Pinkus et al.,[1] solid masses of small basaloid cells grow down from the epidermis (Fig. 2.2). Tumor masses anastomose with each other to create an epithelial network. The tumor stroma is richly vascular and has an angiomatous clinical appearance. The vascular

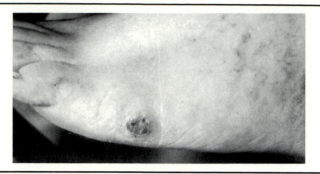

Figure 2.1
Eccrine poroma. A richly vascular nodular growth is revealed after crusts are removed.

stroma is not as well organized in the dermal duct variety (see below). Small cystic spaces may occur within the solid mass, forming a *solid-cystic hidra-denoma.*[5] If the majority of tumor cells are vacuolated or clear, the lesion is a *clear cell hidradenoma* or *eccrine acrospiroma*[6] (Fig. 2.3). If eccrine poroma is found to predominate within the dermis and is composed of various ductal structures with the lumina, it is a *dermal duct tumor*[7] (Fig. 2.4). Dermal duct tumor may be part of a classic eccrine poroma, solid hidradenoma, or acrospiroma. Ductal structures are present in typical eccrine poroma (Fig. 2.2) as well as in the other variants. In contrast to basal cell epithelioma, with which it has been confused, no palisading of tumor cell nuclei at the periphery is observed in typical eccrine poroma or in its variants (Figs. 2.2 and 2.3). The solid masses of strongly basophilic tumor cells are sharply demarcated from surrounding normal epidermis (Fig. 2.2). Intercellular bridges are not as clearly visible between tumor cells as between the squamoid cells of the neighboring epidermis. No sign of keratinization such as squamous eddies or horn pearls is observed. Aggregations of squamoid cells within the tumor represent attempted formation of an acrosyringeal duct (Fig. 2.2B,D). The surface of the lesion is parakeratotic in areas in which the tumor is directly exposed to the surface (Fig. 2.1).

Histochemistry

The presence of glycogen, its synthetic, as well as catabolic enzymes in these tumors support their eccrine differentiation (Fig. 2.5). In normal skin, glycogen is stored in the epidermis, in the outer root sheath of the hair follicle, and in the eccrine gland. However, enzymes involved in glycogen metabolism are present in significant amounts only in the eccrine gland. Glycogen stains such as diastase-labile periodic acid–Schiff (PAS) or silver methenamine stain are positive in the eccrine poromas (Table 1.3). Eccrine-specific monoclonal antikeratin antibody EKH6 labels most of these tumors. Only a sparse focal deposit of CEA was reported in eccrine poroma.[61] S-100 protein is not present in a significant amount.[16]

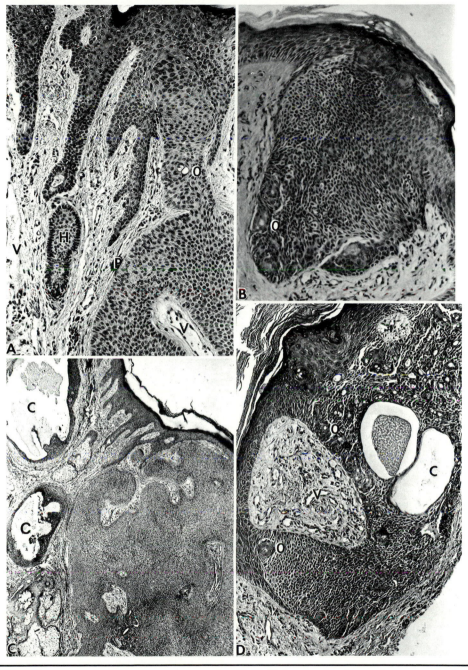

Figure 2.2
Eccrine poroma. In A solid masses of small basaloid cells grow from the epidermis. In contrast to a distinct palisation of hair follicle (H), the peripheral cells of eccrine poroma (P) do not palisade. In B small openings (O) and squamoid wall cells represent ductal differentiation. In C and D large cystic spaces (C) are also formed, producing the picture of solid-cystic hidradenoma. In A and D the stroma contains many capillaries and dilated blood vessels (V). (A and B, × 100; C, × 25; D, × 65.)

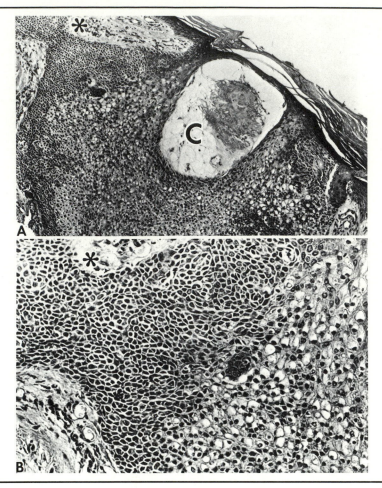

Figure 2.3
Eccrine poroma—clear cell hidradenoma-eccrine acrospiroma. The majority of the cells of this lesion are clear due to their high glycogen content. Peripheral nonpalisading basaloid cells are distinctly poromatous (*). The large cyst (C) is not a glandular differentiation but represents stromal degeneration. (A, × 50 and B, × 150).

Ultrastructure

Ductal lumen formation by coalescence of intracellular cavities is characteristic of eccrine embryonic acrosyringeal duct formation (Table 1.4). These cavities are induced by lytic action of lysosomes. This mode of duct formation has been demonstrated in all the tumors of this group so far examined (Fig. 2.6). Glycogen-rich tumor cells contain a small number of tonofilaments and are connected to each other by poorly developed desmosomes (Fig. 2.7).

Subtypes of Eccrine Poroma

In *eccrine poromatosis*[8,9] numerous papules, sessile lesions, and confluent plaques are present on the soles and palms. In the patient reported by Wilk-

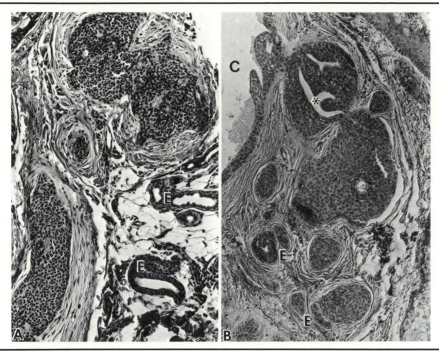

Figure 2.4
Dermal duct tumor. In A the tumor islands are located adjacent to eccrine glands and ducts (E) and are surrounded with fibrous stroma. The lesion in B shows slit-like ductal spaces (*) and a large cyst (C). Small epithelial structures resemble eccrine ducts (E). Fibrous stroma envelopes the lesion. (A and B, × 100.)

inson et al.,[9] closely set, small papular and verrucous lesions were formed on the dorsa of toes, forearms, and calves. Solitary lesions were scattered elsewhere. The patient simultaneously had hidrotic ectodermal dysplasia. The histopathologic picture was identical to that of ordinary eccrine poroma.

Mascaro[10] described *eccrine syringofibroadenoma,* which occurred as a solitary nodular growth in the leg and upper lip of a man and a woman, both 63 years of age. Olmos[11] and Civatte et al.[12] recognized similar tumors. Recently, Mehregan et al.[13] added two more cases, a 78-year-old oriental woman and a 72-year-old Middle Eastern woman, who developed solitary nodular lesions on the foot and wrist respectively. Clinically, these were all benign growths. The histologic picture was characterized by slender, anastomosing epithelial cords forming a sponge-like mass filled in with fibrous and vascular stroma (Fig. 2.8B–D). There was a striking resemblance to the premalignant fibroepithelial tumor of Pinkus[14] except for the presence of ductal structures (Fig. 2.8) and the absence of keratin cysts and small buds of basaloid cells.

In *acrosyringeal nevus* described by Weedon and Lewis[15] (Figs. 2.8A and 2.9), a verrucous plaque 2.5 cm in diameter was found on the dorsum of the hand in a 16-year-old girl; multiple small papules of similar histology developed later on the forearm.[16] In *linear eccrine poroma,* Ogino[17] described a 44-year-old woman in whom numerous brownish red papules extended linearly

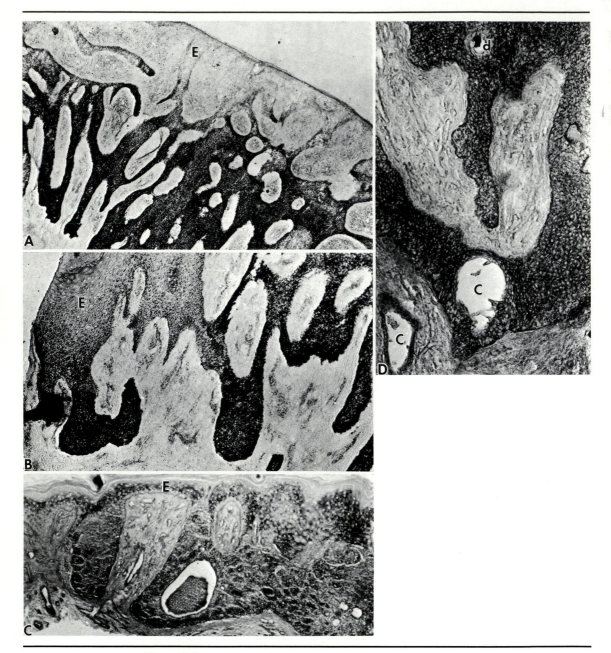

Figure 2.5
Eccrine poroma. Eccrine-dominant enzymes such as succinic dehydrogenase are strongly positive in the anastomosing tumor strand and negative in the normal epidermis (E) that covers the lesion in A and B. Glycogen, demonstrated with PAS stain, is strongly positive in the tumor, as seen in C and D, but is also moderately positive in the epidermis (E in C). Ductal (d) and dilated cystic spaces (C) are seen in D. (A, × 25; B, × 70; C, × 30; D, × 170.)

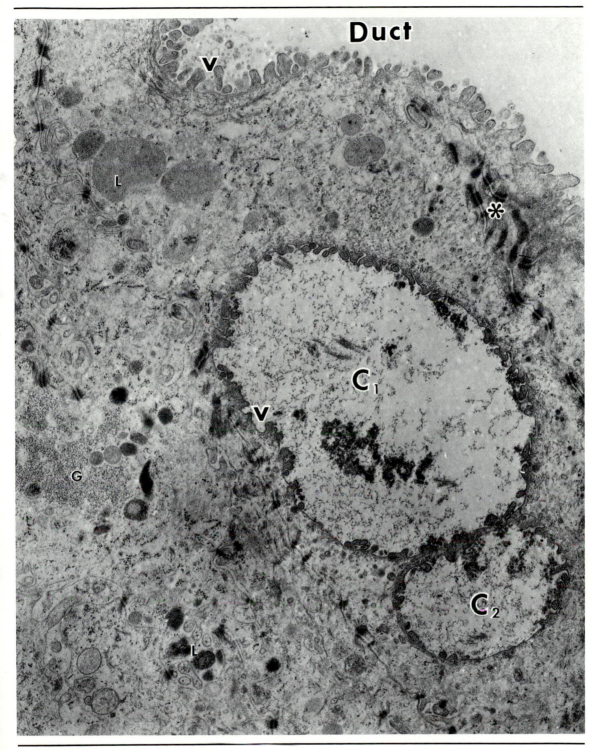

Figure 2.6

Eccrine poroma. Two cavities (C$_1$, C$_2$) are being formed within a luminal cell and are about to merge to make a larger cavity and eventually to communicate with the ductal lumen (Duct). These cavities and duct are lined with the numerous short villi (v) that are typical of ductal differentiation. A chain of closely set desmosomes (∗) seals the intercellular junctions near the duct. G—glycogen particles. L—lysosome. (× 7,000.)

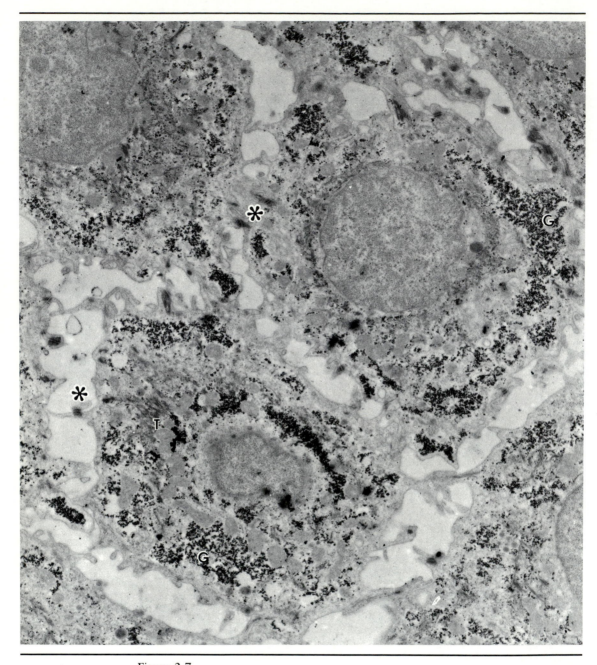

Figure 2.7
Eccrine poroma. The small basophilic tumor cells seen through the light microscope contain a large amount of glycogen (G) and a small number of tonofilaments (T). They are connected by poorly developed desmosomes (*). (× 8,500.)

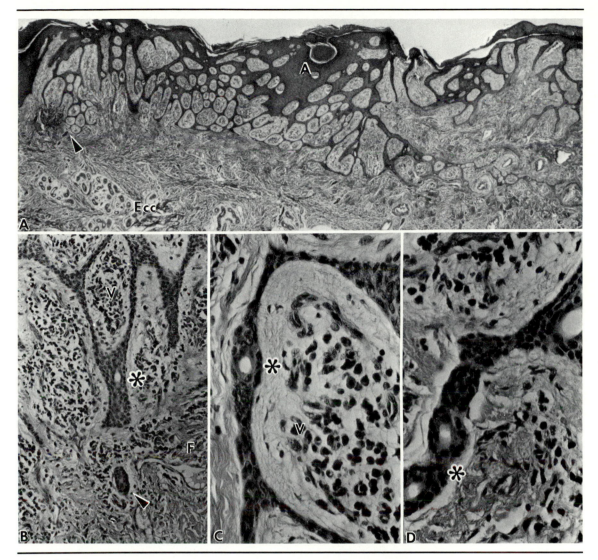

Figure 2.8
*Eccrine syringofibroadenoma, acrosyringeal nevus, or linear eccrine poroma. These
three conditions share similar or identical histology. Thin, anastomosing cords of epithelial networks extend from acanthotic (A) or atrophic epidermis. The stroma is
highly vascular (V) and/or fibrotic (F). Occasionally ductal spaces (*) are found. Eccrine glands (Ecc) are present below the lesion and there is some connection with the
lesion (arrowhead in A and B). The overall picture is very similar to the fibroepithelial tumor of Pinkus. (A, × 33; B, × 163; C and D, × 520.) (Courtesy of David
Weedon, M.D.)*

from foot to thigh, arrayed mostly along the S_2 dermatome of the right leg
except for the lateral aspect of the foot. The lesion had started on the achilles
tendon when she was 24 years old. These two subtypes and eccrine syringofibroadenoma share a common histopathologic feature: in addition to the

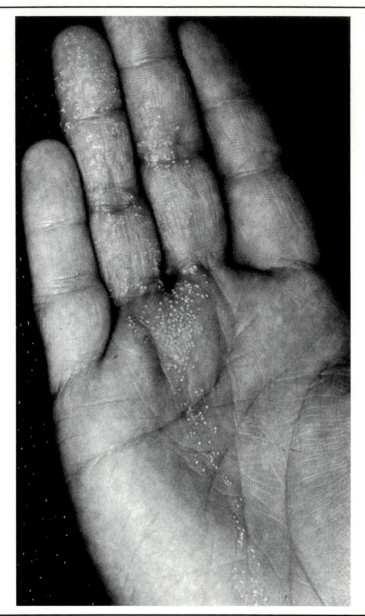

Figure 2.9
Porokeratotic eccrine duct and hair follicle nevus. This linearly arranged erythematous, slightly scaly lesion shows numerous small plugs in the area of the eccrine duct ostia. The lesion extends distally to the ulnar side of his palm and farther to the third and fourth digits. It also extends proximally to the wrist, where follicular plugs are found. (Courtesy of Ralph J. Coskey, M.D.)

typical eccrine poroma-like picture, buds of thin, cord-like strands emerged from the epidermis and anastomosed with each other. These two tumors also resemble the premalignant fibroepithelial tumor of Pinkus[14] except for the presence in the former of occasional ductal lumina.[15,17] Connections with the dermal eccrine ducts were also noted, and there were underlying normal eccrine glands.

In *linear eccrine nevus with comedones* reported by Blanchard et al.,[18] linear comedo-like lesions developed rapidly on the inner aspect of the thigh of a 12-year-old girl. The lesion extended to the ankle. Various tumors were found under the keratotic plugs of the comedones and acanthotic epidermis. Some resembled eccrine spiradenoma and nodular or cystic eccrine hidradenoma; others suggested hyperplastic duct or eccrine dermal duct tumors[7] (Fig. 2.4).

In *porokeratotic eccrine ostial and dermal duct nevus* reported by Abell and Read,[19] linear warty lesions had been present in a 3-year-old girl since birth. The tumors were located on the medial aspect of the great toe and extended proximally across one-third of the left foot on the medial side. Biopsy showed thickened acrosyringium, more squamoid than poroma-like, and the dilated lumen were plugged with cornoid lamellae as in porokeratosis. The dermal duct connected to the lesion was hyperplastic and somewhat resembled a dermal duct tumor, but the underlying eccrine glands were normal. Under the name of *comedo nevus of the palm*, Marsden et al.[20] reported similar comedone-like or pitted linear lesion present on the palm since birth in a 9-year-old boy. Coskey reported with us[21] a case of *porokeratotic eccrine duct and hair follicle nevus*. The patient was a 30-year-old man with a linearly arranged plaque of comedones on one forearm and hand that had been present since the age of 2 years (Fig. 2.10). Thickened acrosyringium on the palm and hair follicles on the wrist were found under the cornoid lamella-like plug (Fig. 2.10). This case was similar to the last two conditions discussed above but shared some features with linear porokeratosis of the hand and foot, whose lesions tend to plug eccrine pores and follicular orifices.[22] Because the thickened acrosyrium is mostly squamoid, as in the normal acrosyringium, and not basaloid, as in eccrine poroma, these three entities may best be regarded as hamartomatous hyperplasia of the acrosyringium and upper dermal duct rather than true poral neoplasia.

Syringoacanthoma of Rahbari[23] is a solitary seborrheic keratosis-like lesion that occurs in various parts of the body and which is predominantly seen in women. Histologically, well-defined clusters of small basophilic cells are present within the substance of an acanthotic and hyperkeratotic epidermis (Fig. 2.11). PAS stain or eccrine-specific monoclonal antibody (Table 1.5) can delineate the mosaicism of the tumor cell nests and surrounding keratinocytes. An eccrine duct may lead into the lesion, and ductal lumina may be found within the tumor nests. This tumor may be regarded as a variant of eccrine poroma or hidroacanthoma simplex (see below) in which an acanthotic and papillomatous reaction of the epidermal keratinocytes occurs. In *malignant syringoacanthoma*, dysplastic acrosyringeal cells that are hyperchromatic and irregular in size and shape (atypia) intermingle with the epidermal keratinocytes, and dermal invasion may be present[21,23] (Fig. 2.12).

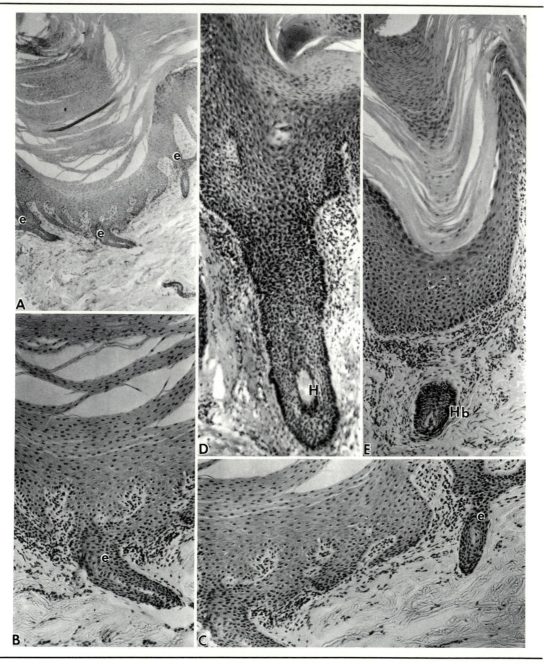

Figure 2.10
Porokeratotic eccrine duct and hair follicle nevus. In A through C eccrine duct ori-
fices (e) are plugged with a column of parakeratotic keratin. In D and E the follicu-
lar orifice is also plugged with a piled mass of parakeratotic cells. H—hair. Hb—
hair bulb. A, × 33; B and C, × 65; D and E, × 100.) (Courtesy of Ralph J. Cos-
key, M.D.)

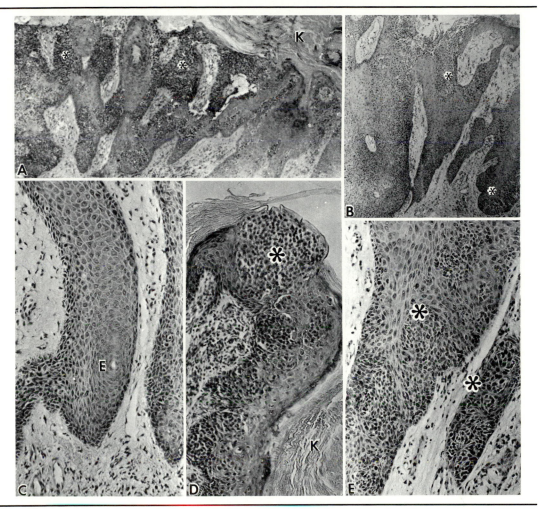

Figure 2.11
Syringoacanthoma. A markedly hyperkeratotic (K) and acanthotic epidermis contains multiple ill-defined islands of small basaloid cells (*) that are similar to eccrine poroma (see Fig. 2.2) or dermal duct tumor (see Fig. 2.4). Some elongated rete ridges contain eccrine sweat ducts (E). (A, × 22; B, × 52; C, D, and E, × 163.) (Courtesy of Homayoon Rahbari, M.D.)

Hidroacanthoma simplex[24,25] is an intraepidermal form of eccrine poroma. It occurs predominantly in women and arises in the extremities as a hyperkeratotic plaque resembling seborrheic keratosis or Bowen's disease. Intraepidermal nests vary in size but may occupy large areas (Fig. 2.13). The small cuboidal tumor cells contain glycogen. The poromatous growth may contain duct-like slit or round lumen. A few dendritic melanocytes may be present. Seborrheic keratosis with intraepidermal nests may resemble this entity; however, in seborrheic keratosis the small basaloid cells do not contain glycogen.

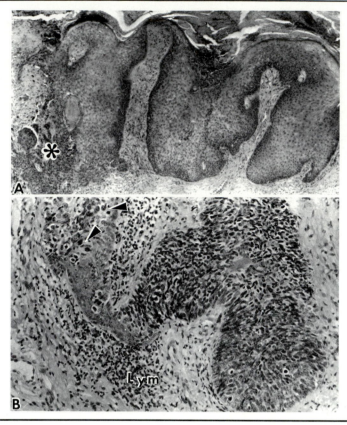

Figure 2.12
Malignant syringoacanthoma. This lesion is beginning to break through the base-
ment membrane (*). Tumor cells are hyperchromatic and polymorphic and are gen-
erally larger (arrowheads in B) than those of a benign variety (see Fig. 2.11).
Separation of these cells from surrounding keratinocytes by nest formation is less
distinct. Lymphocyte infiltrate (Lym), a defense mechanism, is heavy in these areas
of tumor invasion. (A, × 22 and B, × 163.) (Courtesy of Homayoon Rahbari,
M.D.)

The so-called Borst-Jadassohn intraepidermal epithelioma does not exist as a single entity. Borst's patient had an invasive squamous cell carcinoma with foci of anaplastic cells extending into the surrounding epidermis.[26] On rare occasions we encounter well-circumscribed aggregations of squamoid cells that do not belong to actinic keratosis or Bowen's disease (Fig. 2.14A). Jadassohn described a lesion that was most likely a seborrheic keratosis with intraepidermal nest formation[27] (Fig. 2.14B). Other lesions that form intraepidermal islands of tumor cells include hidroacanthoma simplex and syringoacanthoma,[23,24] or lesions that are not typical of either but have irregularly shaped aggregations of basaloid cells (Fig. 2.14C).

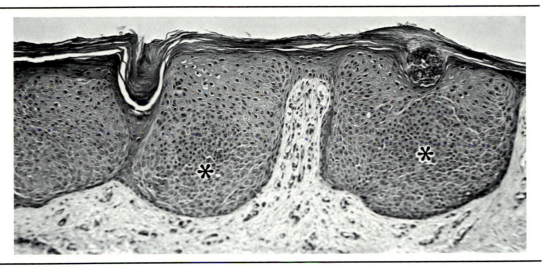

Figure 2.13
Hidroacanthoma simplex. Aggregations of small basaloid cells (∗) are found in the epidermis. (× 150.)

Eccrine Porocarcinoma (Malignant Eccrine Poroma)

Approximately half of eccrine adenocarcinomas are of this variety.[28–31] The lesion may present as a localized nodule, a plaque, or an ulcerated tumor, commonly located on the extremities and head in elderly individuals.[32] Extensive lymphatic spread into the surrounding skin and distant metastasis may occur. Histologically, the skin metastasis tends to be epidermotropic and resembles Paget's disease.[28,29]

Histology

The malignant epithelial tumor masses show irregularly shaped cells with hyperchromatic nuclei and multinucleated giant cells. Intraepidermal islands of anaplastic cells may be present on top of the dermal lesion (Fig. 2.15). In some tumors eosinophilic squamoid rather than basophilic basaloid cells predominate (Fig. 2.15E, F). Either part of the tumor, or the majority of some tumors are composed of basaloid and anaplastic squamoid cells (Fig. 2.15C, E). Many vacuolated cells undergoing duct formation (Fig. 2.15E, F) or well-formed ducts are encountered (Fig. 2.15E). Atypia, pleomorphism, and mitotic figures are common. Tumor cells of some cases of extramammary Paget's disease or porocarcinoma are PAS positive; however, the former is diastase resistant (because of the presence of sialomucin) while the latter is diastase labile (because of glycogen).

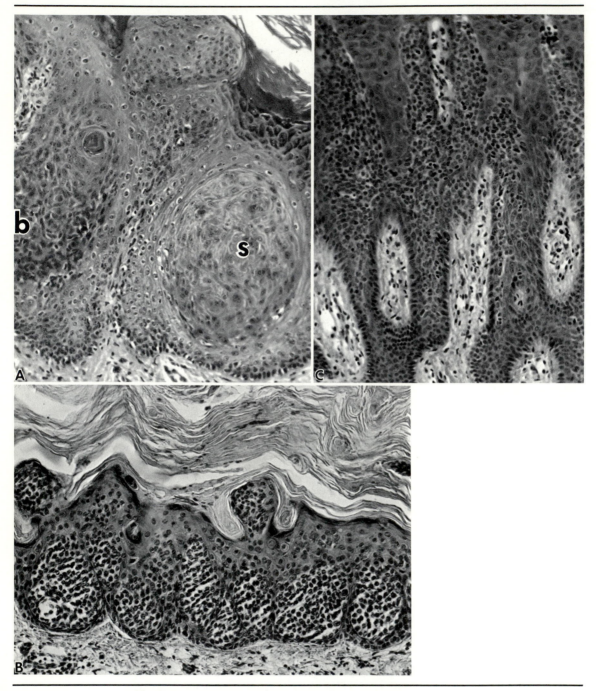

Figure 2.14
Intraepidermal epithelioma. In A squamoid cells (s) make nests in the center; basaloid cells also form nests (b). This lesion resembles irritated seborrheic keratosis. In B the lesion resembles a clonal type of seborrheic keratosis. In C a syringoacanthoma-like lesion without ductal differentiation is shown. (A, B and C, × 170.) (A and C courtesy of Martin C. Mihm, Jr., M.D.)

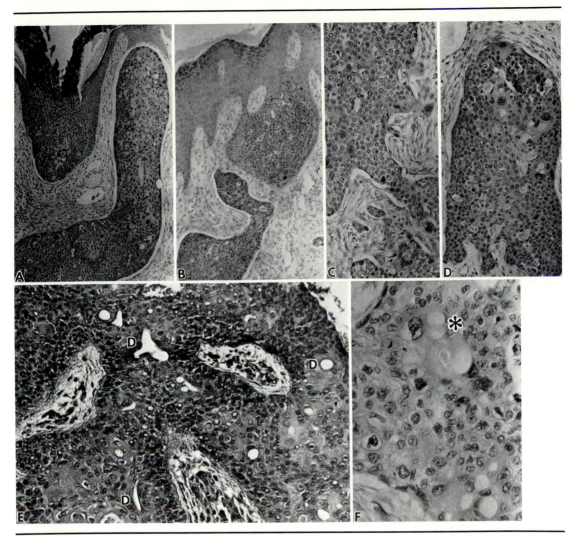

Figure 2.15
*Malignant eccrine poroma or porocarcinoma. In A and B epithelial strands grow
down from the epidermis, anastomose to each other, and form a network. In C and
D two types of cells, poroma-like basaloid cells at the periphery, and squamoid giant
cells with nuclear hyperchromasia and atypia, are seen near the center of the strands.
In E and F evidence of duct formation is seen in vacuolated cells (*) and well-
formed ducts (D) in round or slit-like profile. (A, × 29; B, × 47; C, D, and E, ×
117; F, × 450.)*

Clear Cell Hidradenoma (Eccrine Acrospiroma)

Other names used to designate this tumor include clear cell myoepithelioma, solid-cystic hidradenoma, hidradenocarcinoma, large cell sweat gland adenoma, and porosyringoma, among others. It is usually a single, solid nodule 1 to 2 cm in diameter and covered with normal skin. It may be cystic, and the covering skin may be red, blue, thickened, and even papillated.[33] About 16% of the lesions show drainage and about the same number are painful.[34] Clear fluid may be discharged upon surgical incision. There is no predilection site.

Histology

The lesion arises as an encapsulated or nonencapsulated, multilobulated tumor in the dermis.[35] If it is large, compressed collagen bundles become hyalinized and may form a pseudocapsule (Fig. 2.16). The tumor is sometimes connected to the epidermis. Such tumors resemble eccrine poroma or eccrine dermal duct tumors except that they contain a large number of vacuolated or clear cells which are larger and more eosinophilic, even in the solid part. However, features of eccrine poroma often coexist (see Fig. 2.3). It is best to regard this tumor as part of the spectrum of eccrine acrosyringium—eccrine duct proliferation. Abundant eccrine-type enzymes are present.[36,37] Ultrastructurally, clear cell hidradenoma shares the features of both eccrine dermal duct tumors and acrosyringium. A small number of tumor cells resemble eccrine secretory cells.[36]

The tumor cells are round, fusiform, or polygonal. The glycogen-rich vacuolated (clear) cells have a distinct cell wall and often an eccentrically displaced nucleus (Fig. 2.16C). Slit-like spaces are present and lined by a layer of cuboidal cells resembling an eccrine dermal duct. Whorls of large squamoid cells with a central cavity may be found embedded in the parenchyma; these mimic intraepidermal ducts. Small aggregates of clear cells form vacuoles in some tumors; these could be interpreted as abortive attempts to form ductal structures (Fig. 2.16B). In other tumors, cystic spaces and ductal structures are abundant; these lesions could be called solid-cystic hidradenomas[27] (Fig. 2.17).

Syringoma

This tumor, although located in the superficial dermis,[38] represents a differentiation toward eccrine acrosyringium. There are several clinical varieties.

The *eyelid type* is the most common and classic presentation. The lower eyelids are usually more involved (Fig. 2.18A). Fawn-colored, grain-sized, globoid papules are slightly elevated but asymptomatic. The onset is usually at puberty, and new lesions continue to appear until middle age.

Eruptive syringoma or eruptive hidradenoma[39] is a less common variety affecting younger individuals, including children. Discrete or confluent pap-

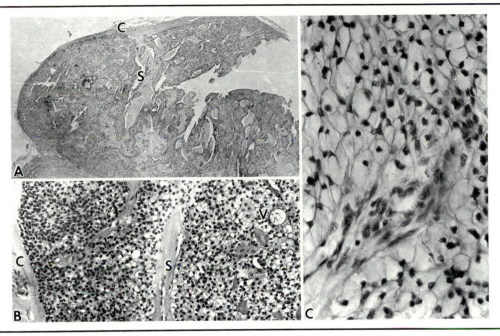

Figure 2.16
*Clear cell hidradenoma or acrospiroma. A large tumor is encapsulated (C) with hy-
alinized collagen bundles that extend into the parenchyma as septae (S) and divide it
into many lobules (A and B). The parenchyma consists of small basophilic or poromatous cells and larger clear cells. Primitive intraepidermal or acrosyringeal types of
duct formation are seen in a group of several vacuolated cells (V). (A, × 22; B, ×
65; C, × 163.)*

ules with the same characteristics as the eyelid type occur diffusely over the
anterior half of the body and flexor side of the upper arms. A heavy concentration of papular lesions is seen on the anterior neck and upper chest (Fig.
2.18B, C). The predominant distribution pattern of the lesion over the anterior
half of the body may correspond to a generally denser distribution of the
eccrine gland over the anterior side of the body. The umbilical area and lower
abdomen may be heavily involved (Fig. 2.18D, E). Rarely, cases of this type[40]
as well as the eyelid variety[41] are familial.

   Localized syringomas other than the eyelid type also occur. Syringoma can
be limited to the vulva[42] or penis[43] (genital syringoma) or to the dorsum of
the fingers[44] (acral syringoma). It may be unilateral or linear in distribution,[45]
similar to systematized epidermal nevus. When it occurs in the scalp, it may
be associated with cicatricial alopecia.[46–48] Very rare varieties include lesions
with a bathing trunk distribution[49] or unilateral tumors.[50] Some cases initially
show limited distribution but later spread widely, typically taking the form of
eruptive syringoma. A few cases of very late onset are on record.[51] A significant number of cases are associated with Down's syndrome.[52–54] Occurrence
with Marfan's or Ehlers–Danlos syndromes[54] may be fortuitous.

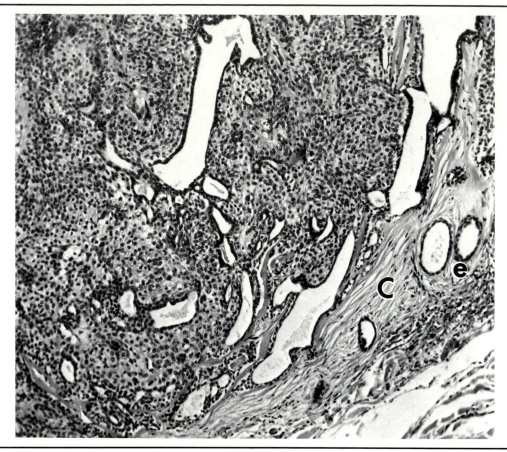

Figure 2.17
Clear cell hidradenoma or solid cystic hidradenoma. Although predominantly cystic, solid areas consist of both basophilic and clear cells. The capsule (C) contains a few dilated eccrine ducts (e). The cystic spaces are lined with one layer of dense cuboidal cells, most likely eccrine ductal epithelium. (× 140.) (Courtesy of Martin C. Mihm, Jr., M.D.)

Histology

All three clinical types of syringoma share the same histologic features. Small, round to ovoid epithelial masses, with or without lumen, are found in the superficial dermis and resemble oblique sections of eccrine duct (Fig. 2.19). A short cord of epithelial cells with a tadpole shape is often attached (Fig. 2.19B). Large cystic cavities with keratin sheaths may be found, sometimes connected to the epidermal rete ridges (Fig. 2.19A). Some lesions contain excessive cystic spaces within the epithelial mass produced by coalescence of multiple vesicles and vacuoles (Fig. 2.20A) as the eccrine acrosyringeal duct is formed in fetal life.[55] Some tumors are primarily ductal and resemble eccrine dermal ducts (Fig. 2.20B). The cysts contain eosinophilic material that is PAS positive and diastase resistant (Figs. 2.19B, C and 2.20C). Electron microscopy reveals that

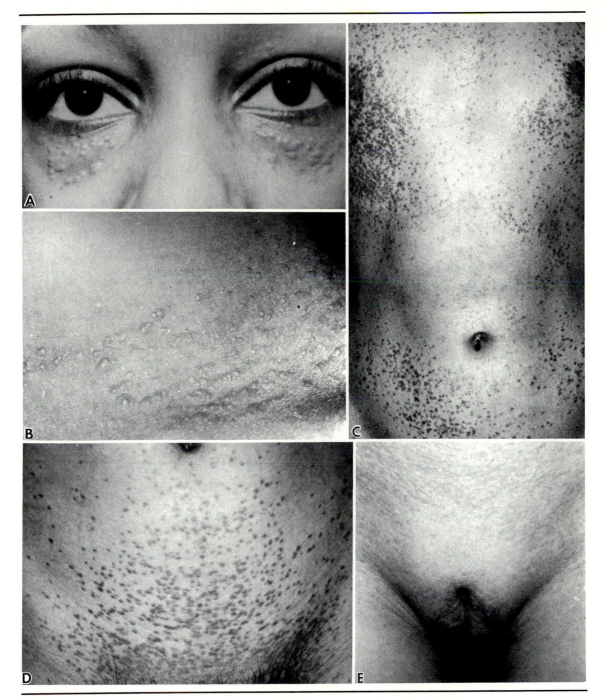

Figure 2.18
Syringoma of lower eyelids (A) and eruptive syringoma (hidradenoma) of anterior
neck (B), anterior trunk (C), and lower abdomen (D and E). Individual lesions are
small fawn-colored papules (A). They may become confluent and form plaques (C),
or arrange themselves in continuous linear fashion along the cleavage line of the skin
(B).

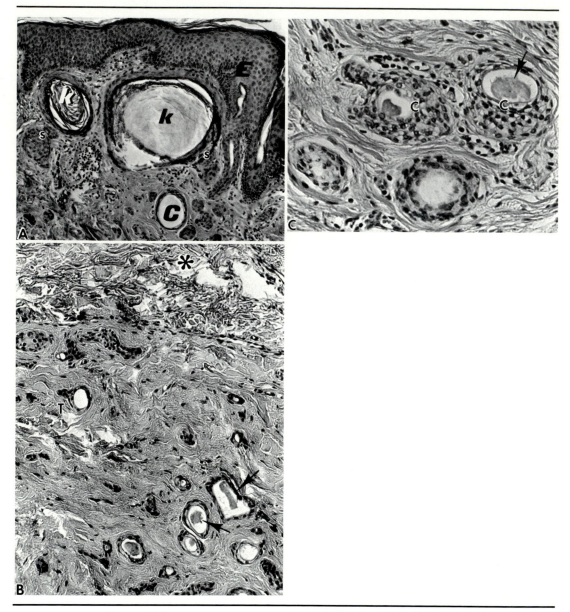

Figure 2.19
Syringoma. In A, a cystic lesion (c) is connected to an eccrine duct (E). Large keratin-filled cysts (k) are located just under the epidermis: these may be attached to epithelial islands of syringoma (s). In B, small cystic lesions and solid epithelial nests and cords are embedded in a sclerotic stroma that is distinctly different from the surrounding loose connective tissue (*) seen below the epidermis. Some cysts are attached by a short epithelial cord to form a "tadpole" cyst (T). Large cysts contain eosinophilic substance (arrows) that is a neutral mucopolysaccharide (PAS positive, diastase resistant). In C, a thick epithelial wall of some cysts (C) is composed of large, clear cells, thus resembling clear cell syringoma (see Fig. 2.21). (A and B, × 45; C, × 65.)

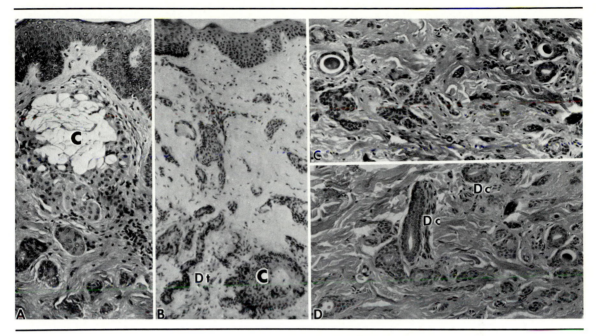

Figure 2.20
Syringoma. In A *and* B *within a mass of epithelial cells, multiple vacuoles are produced and a large cyst (C) is formed by their coalescence. Some structures are distinctly ductal given their elongated tubular configuration (Dt) or by the presence of a cuticular border (Dc). Hyalinized sclerotic stroma is evident in* A, C, *and* D. (A, C, *and* D, × 43; B, × 24.)

this material is composed of numerous vesicles and lysosomes (see Fig. 2.25). In *clear cell syringoma*, a large amount of glycogen fills the tumor cells and causes them to appear empty (clear)[56,57] (Fig. 2.21). A transitional lesion between the solid epithelial variety and the totally clear cell type may be seen (Fig. 2.19C). Under the title *eccrine centered nevus*,[58] Mishima reported grouped papules of intradermal nevus ensheathing a normal eccrine duct; Schellander et al.[59] described a single lesion on the bridge of the nose that consisted of both syringoma and intradermal nevus.

The stroma in syringoma contains a large number of mast cells. In some instances, as reported by Seifert,[60] the clinical picture is one of disseminated lesions of urticaria pigmentosa. Epithelial or ductal lesions are embedded in a fibrous stroma of their own (Figs. 2.19 and 2.20).

Histochemistry
All eccrine type enzymes (Figs. 2.22 and 2.23) and eccrine substances (Table 1.3), including glycogen on PAS stain, are positive.[38] Eccrine-specific monoclonal antibody EKH6 (Fig. 2.24B, C, D, E) labels the luminal border of ductal and cystic lesions, while basal cell-specific monoclonal antikeratin antibody

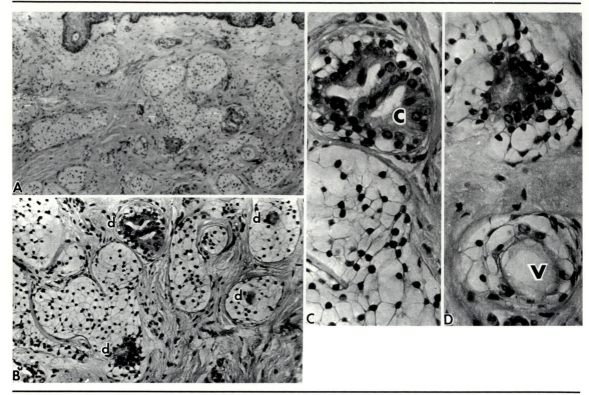

Figure 2.21
*Clear cell syringoma. In A and B aggregation of clear cells or islands of various sizes
are seen in the dermis. In B, C, and D some clear cell islands show typical eccrine
ductal structures (d) with an eosinophilic cuticle (C) or multivacuolated center (V),
the latter being the process of primordial cavity formation of acrosyringeal duct. (A,
× 15; B, × 25; C and D, × 160.) (Courtesy of Peter J. Aronson, M.D.)*

EKH4 stains the outer layers of epithelial cords and cyst walls (Fig. 2.24A).
EKH5, another monoclonal antibody that labels eccrine secretory epithelium,
is entirely negative in this lesion. S100 protein, an acidic calcium-binding
protein originally isolated from the brain, is present in eccrine secretory segments but not in the duct.[61] Syringoma has no S100 protein by immunohistochemistry.[61] These data support the ultrastructural findings that the tumor
differentiates toward eccrine duct in or near the acrosyringium.

Electron Microscopy

The ductal and cystic borders are lined with typical ductal epithelium, bearing
on its surface short but numerous luminal villi. In addition, these luminal cells
contain a large number of multivesicular bodies and electron-dense granules,
that is, lysosomes (Fig. 2.25A, B) and occasionally, keratohyaline granules[38]
(Fig. 2.25C). In areas of active cyst or lumen formation, as depicted in Fig.

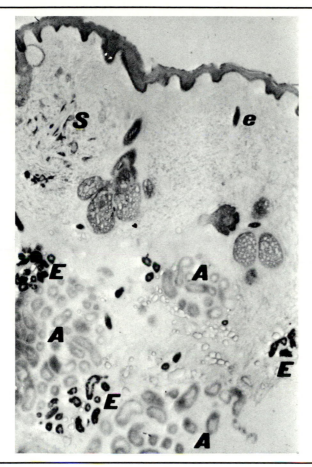

Figure 2.22
Syringoma. Amylophosphorylase is strongly positive in the syringoma lesion (S), the eccrine secretory segment (E), and the eccrine duct (e) but is negative in the apocrine gland (A); thus a similarity is seen between syringoma and eccrine structures. (× 25.)

2.20A, digestion of cytoplasm by these lysosomes and multiple cavity formation are observed (Fig. 2.25A). In large keratinous cysts that are usually connected to the epidermis or rete ridges (Fig. 2.19A) keratohyalin granules are large and numerous. These luminal cells undergo mostly incomplete keratinization, as observed in the acrosyringeal duct near the skin surface.[38,62] (Fig. 2.25C).

Chondroid Syringoma

In this neoplasm the fibrous tumor stroma shows areas of chondroid metaplasia. The lesion, also called mixed tumor of the skin of eccrine or salivary

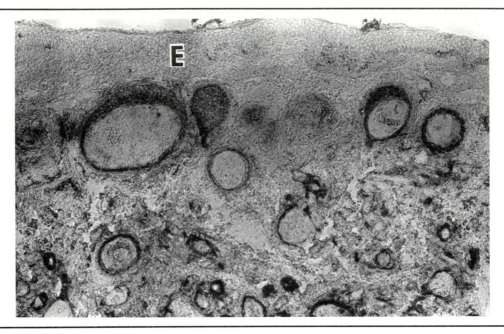

Figure 2.23
Syringoma. Succinic dehydrogenase is strongly positive in the epithelial masses, cords, and cyst walls. The epidermis (E) is nonreactive. (× 65.)

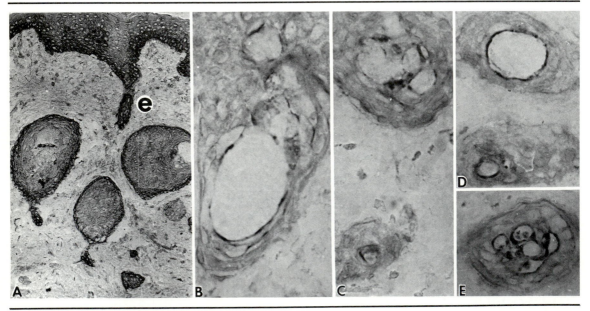

Figure 2.24
Syringoma. EKH4, which recognizes basal cell keratin, also stains the periphery of the syringoma lesion and the eccrine duct (e) in A. EKH6, which labels the eccrine gland and duct, stains the luminal keratin in B, C, D, and E. The immunoperoxidase method is used. (A, × 50; B, C, D, and E, × 520.)

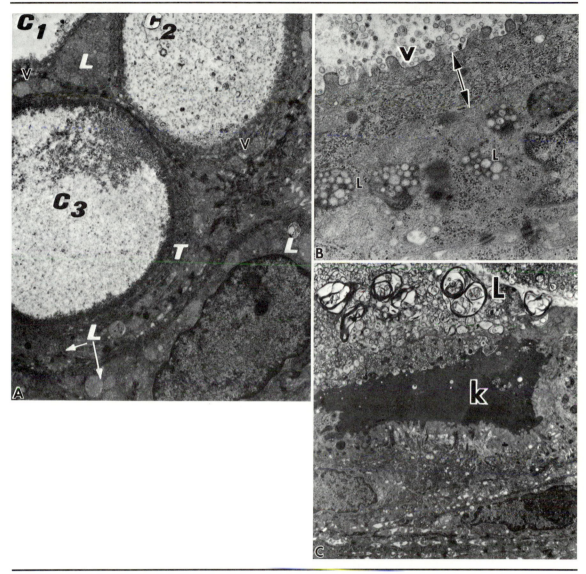

Figure 2.25

Syringoma. In A the luminal cells of three primordial cystic cavities (C₁, C₂, C₃) bear numerous short villi (v). Along the luminal border a tonofilament-rich zone (T) is recognized. These are all ductal features. This cell also contains lysosomes of a multivesicular dense body type (L), seen in embryonic production of eccrine intraepidermal ducts. In B the luminal villi (V), the periluminal filamentous zone (between arrows), and the multivesicular dense bodies (L) are enlarged. In C a completely keratinized cell (k) lines the lumen as in the midportion of the eccrine intraepidermal duct. The lumen (L) contains vesicles derived from the lysosomes of luminal cells and myelin figured membrane debris. (A and C, × 5,000; B, × 58,500.)

gland type, occurs most commonly in the head and neck region.[63] Clinically, both types are firm intracutaneous nodules covered with normal epidermis. A rare malignant variety tends to occur in the extremities and is malignant from the start. It shows a wide range of malignant manifestations,[64–67] from local recurrences to fatal distant metastasis.

Histology

It is more practical to consider epithelial components and stromal variations separately than to classify each tumor into tubulocystic type, with branching lumina, small tubular lumen type,[68–71] etc. These subtypes overlap substantially and many variations and combinations are seen, even within the same tumor. The eccrine and salivary types show the same histologic picture.

Epithelial variations (Figs. 2.26 and 2.27) include the presence of solid masses; thin cords or nests of basaloid cells; tubulocystic areas resembling syringoma (Fig. 2.27B); epithelial masses with large numbers of clear cells that could easily be mistaken for, or indeed be identical to, clear cell hidradenoma (Fig. 2.26D); apocrine-like large lumen formation with columnar epithelium (Fig. 2.27A); pilar differentiation including pilomatricoma; keratin cysts and epithelial nests (Fig. 2.26F), as in trichoepithelioma; meningothelial whorls; scattered single cells with halos identical to chondrocytes (Fig. 2.26A, C, E, F); and melanocytes.[63] The stroma may be fibrous, myxoid, chondroid, hyalin, osseous, or adipoid[63] (Figs. 2.26, 2.27). Chondrocyte-like cells with halo are actually true chondrocytes and satisfy all fine structural criteria for this cell type.[68,72] Mucinous or myxoid stroma (Fig. 2.27B) contains sulfated acid mucopolysaccharide (chondroitin sulfate), and thus will stain with alcian blue but resists hyaluronidase.[73] Stroma is stained metachromatically with toluidine blue or Giemsa. Hyalinized areas are PAS positive and diastase resistant. The parenchyma is EKH 5 and 6 reactive.

Malignant chondroid syringoma shows a marked nuclear pleomorphism, increased mitotic figures, more solid strands of basaloid cells, and less tubular differentiation.[67]

Histogenesis

Based upon electron microscopic studies and a colony-forming assay, Mills[63,68] proposed a monoclonal matrix cell theory. He found "ambivalent" cells with epithelial features (desmosomes, tonofilaments) as well as mesenchymal elements (rough endoplasmic reticulum, Golgi, and basement membrane). Progeny of a single tumor cell, that is, a monoclonal cell line, differentiated into heterogeneous colonies showing epithelial, mesenchymal, and ambivalent cells in close association.[69] It has been thought that myoepithelial cells extending from the tubulocystic epithelium produce a chondroid matrix.[70] However, electron microscopy revealed only a small number of myoepithelial cells surrounding well-formed epithelial nests and ducts.[63] A colony-forming assay did not differentiate myoepithelial cells.[69] The monoclonal theory of Mills[63,68] is diametrically opposed to that of Hirsch and Helwig.[73] They proposed that the tumor is primarily an epithelial one with secondary changes in the stroma.

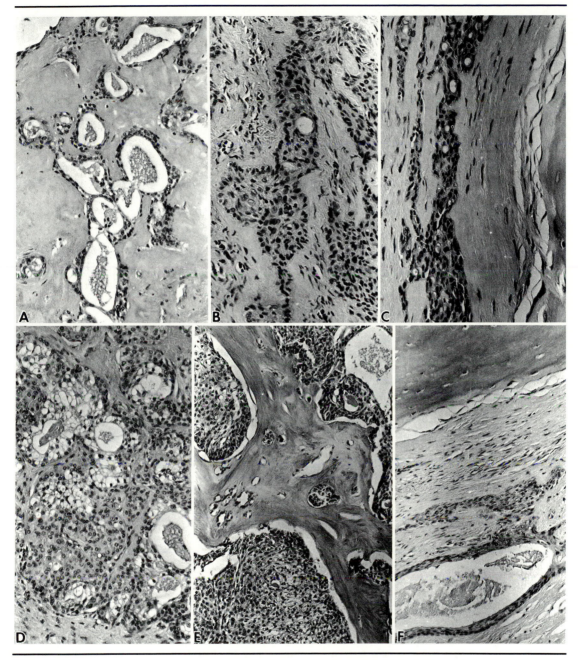

Figure 2.26
*Chondroid syringoma. Embedded in a sclerotic or chondroid stroma one finds
syringoma-like cystic spaces (A), solid basaloid cell areas (B), epithelial cords with
small duct-like spaces (C), clear cell area (D and E), and keratin or hair follicle cysts
(F). (A through F, × 163.)*

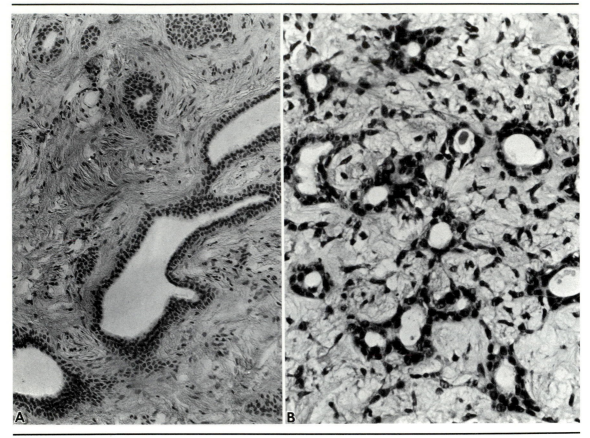

Figure 2.27
Chondroid syringoma. Large luminal spaces are lined with tall columnar cells (A); these glands are similar to apocrine secretory segments. In B syringoma-like or ec-crine gland-like structures are embedded in mucinous stroma. (A, × 130; B, × 163.)

Eccrine Hidrocystoma or Cystadenoma

This tumor or cyst is a dilation of the eccrine dermal (straight) duct, that is, the portion between the coiled duct and the acrosyringium. Although multiple lesions may be produced by acute and chronic exposure to heat (Fig. 2.28), such as a cook receives to the face, our experience, like Smith and Chernosky's,[74] indicates that most lesions are solitary. The male to female ratio is nearly equal. In some patients with numerous lesions, the number of cysts increases in warm weather and decreases in winter.[75,76] Individual lesions may be visible as semitranslucent small facial nodules with a slightly bluish color similar to the apocrine hidrocystoma. More frequently, the cyst is a palpable intradermal nodule covered by normal skin.

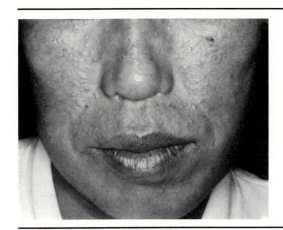

Figure 2.28
Eccrine hidrocystoma. After an acute heat exposure multiple small papules and intradermal nodules developed on the face.

Histology
The large, dilated cyst is seen in the middermis often surrounded with hemorrhagic foci (Fig. 2.29B). This may indicate that the duct was dilated under pressure, causing damage to the surrounding connective tissue. In contrast to syringoma, a well-organized fibrous stroma is rare; the stroma is rather edematous and may consist only of a thin rim of compressed or hyalinized collagen directly outside the cyst wall (Fig. 2.29E, F). The cyst wall is typically double layered (Fig. 2.29D, E) but occasionally may be atrophic and consist of a single flat layer. In some lesions it is hypertrophic with papillary tuft formation (Fig. 2.29D, F). Squamous metaplasia may occur in some parts of the wall. Serial sections demonstrate the connection to the underlying eccrine duct (Fig. 2.29B and E) but seldom to the acrosyringium, where the occlusion may have originated.

Histochemistry
Eccrine types of enzymes such as phosphorylase and succinic dehydrogenase were demonstrated by Ebner and Erlach.[76]

Electron Microscopy
The luminal cells are of a ductal type[77] in that they bear numerous luminal villi and have many desmosomal junctions but lack secretory (mucous) granules (Fig. 2.30) (Table 1.4). Absence of myoepithelial cells rules out the possibility that the tumor is differentiating into a secretory segment of the eccrine gland.

Papillary Eccrine Adenoma

This is a more adenomatous variety of eccrine ductal tumor than is eccrine hidrocystoma, in which papillary tufts may be seen only occasionally. Since

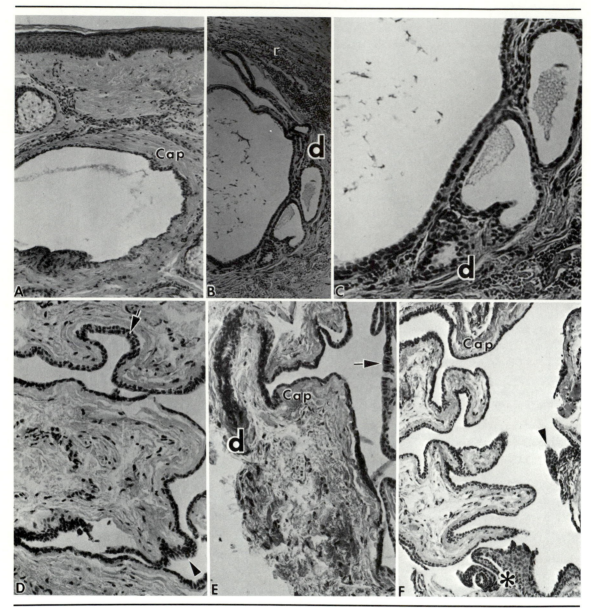

Figure 2.29
Eccrine hidrocystoma. A large simple cyst (A), a large cyst with associated dilated eccrine ducts (d) in the vicinity (B, C, and E), multiply infolding cyst wall (D, E, and F) and papillomatous growth of the wall (arrowheads in D and F) are seen. One part of the wall in F shows squamoid metaplasia (*). Two rows of wall cells are cuboidal in the outer (basal) row and cylindrical in the inner (luminal) layer (arrows in D and E). Connective tissue surrounding the cyst is either sclerotic (Cap in A, E, and F), hemorrhagic (r in B) or edematous (F). (A, B, and F, × 65; C, × 200; D and E, × 130.)

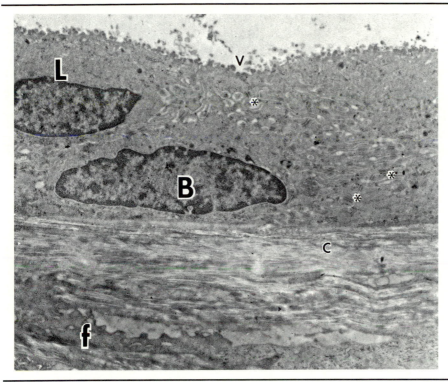

Figure 2.30
Eccrine hidrocystoma. The wall of the cyst consists of two layers of epithelial cells; the basal or outer cells (B) and the luminal or inner cells (L) are essentially the same and are connected to each other with desmosomes (*). The luminal cells differentiate numerous short villi (v) along their luminal border. Compressed collagen bundles (C) surrounding the basal cells correspond to the hyalinized capsule (see Fig. 2.29 A, E, F). f—fibroblast. (× 8,000.)

the first description by Rulon and Helwig in 1977,[78] a few other reports[79–81] have followed. Hands and feet are common sites. It is usually a solitary nodular lesion and may recur.

Histopathology

The well-circumscribed tumor shows cystic, dilated, and branching ductal structures. The wall may be composed of flattened outer and inner cells resembling an eccrine duct; in other areas the wall epithelium is thickened and protrudes into the cystic lumen to form papillary projections (Fig. 2.31). There may be underlying eccrine glands, and some portion of this tumor seems to be differentiated into eccrine glandular adenoma (Fig. 2.31B). The tumor spectrum thus ranges from ductal adenoma, which could be regarded as a syringoma or an eccrine hidrocystoma with intraluminal papillary proliferation, to

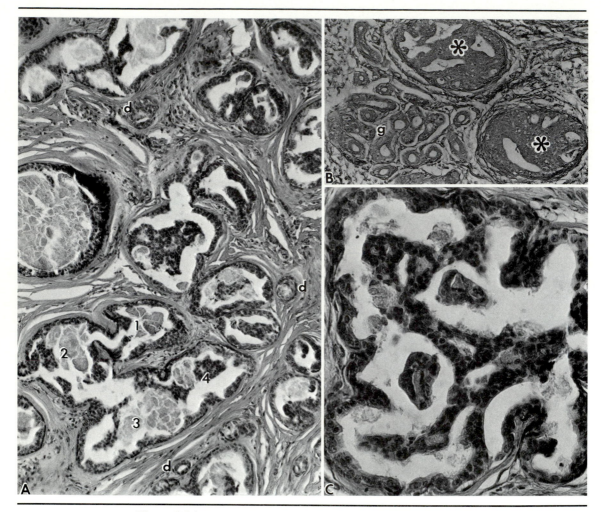

Figure 2.31
*Papillary eccrine adenoma. In A, dilated ductal spaces and cysts are seen. The walls
of these cysts form papillary projections into the lumen. Typical eccrine ducts (d)
seen in the vicinity may be continuous with the lesions. In B some lesions or part of
the lesions show a glandular (*) rather than a ductal adenoma. Normal eccrine
glands (g) are found in the vicinity. In A and C large cystic structures may be produced by coalescence of smaller ones (1, 2, 3, 4 in A). (A, × 180; B, × 130; C, ×
250.)*

an eccrine gland adenoma of the secretory type. Eccrine-specific antikeratin
antibodies EKH6 (gland and duct) (Fig. 2.32) and EKH5 (gland) have been
positive in two cases. The apocrine equivalent of papillary eccrine adenoma
is tubular apocrine adenoma.[82] It is sometimes difficult to differentiate the
two except that decapitation secretion is more prominent in the apocrine
variety.

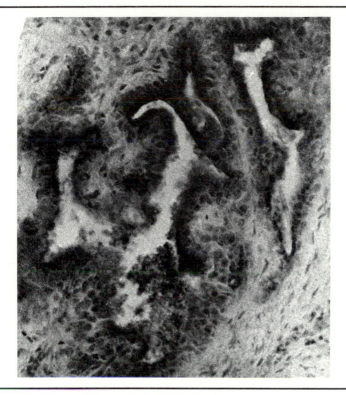

Figure 2.32
Papillary eccrine adenoma. Monoclonal eccrine type antikeratin antibody EKH6 labeled papillary wall cells strongly and specifically. (× 250.)

Aggressive Digital Papillary Adenoma

This tumor has some features that overlap with papillary eccrine adenoma. Fingers and toes and the adjacent skin of the palms and soles are the reported sites.[83] Patients ranged in age from 26 to 66 years with a median age of 44 in Graham's series.[83] The lesion tends to infiltrate deep tissue and recurred in one-third of the cases; the recurrent lesion showed significant cellular atypia.[84] These recurrent lesions are classified as aggressive digital papillary adenocarcinoma. At least 40% of the recurrent lesions had regional lymph node and/or pulmonary metastasis.[84]

Histology

In relatively benign areas or lesions, eccrine ductal and glandular structures are maintained, and the tumor resembles papillary eccrine adenoma (Figs. 2.33 and 2.34). In the adenocarcinomatous area of the tumor or variety, the tumor is more cellular, less glandular, and is pleomorphic. Mitotic figures are frequent (Fig. 2.34D, E, F).

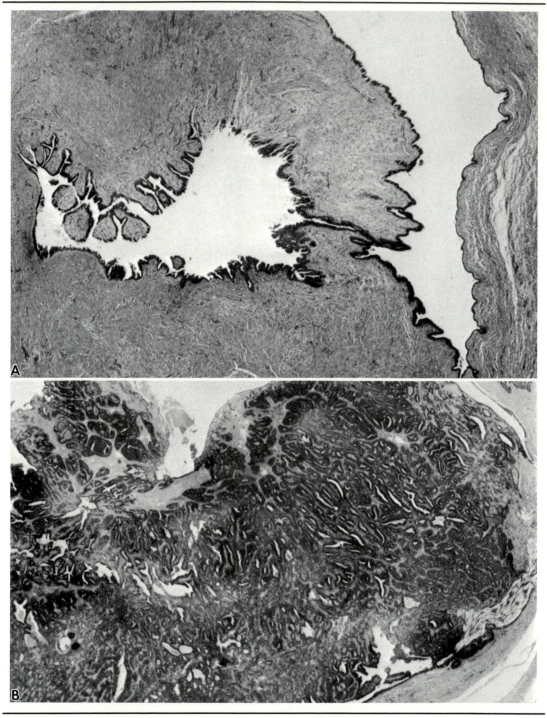

Figure 2.33
Aggressive digital papillary adenoma and adenocarcinoma. In A, many papillary villi project into cystic spaces. In B, glandular areas are composed of entangled cords of eccrine gland-like adenoma. More malignant areas or tumors are cellular rather than glandular. (A and B, × 65.) (Courtesy of David Weedon, M.D.)

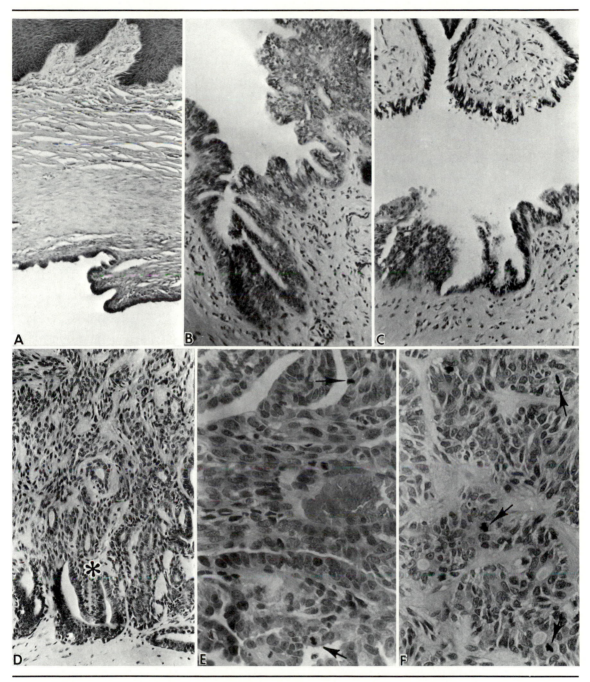

Figure 2.34
Aggressive digital papillary adenoma and adenocarcinoma. Adenomatous or glandular portions and solid cellular areas are seen in the cyst wall in A, B, and C. Glandular structures are predominant in D; even very cellular masses contain some ductal components (in D). Malignant features such as multinucleated giant cells, nuclear hyperchromatism, and frequent mitosis (arrows) are seen in E and F. (A, × 80; B and C, × 130; D, E, and F, × 163.) (Courtesy of David Weedon, M.D.)*

Eccrine Spiradenoma

This is one of the least mature eccrine tumors. It may show some features of eccrine ductal and secretory epithelium. In such cases the presence of tubular ducts with numerous luminal villi suggests ductal differentiation, while the presence of myoepithelial cells indicates differentiation toward the secretory segment of the eccrine gland. The tumor is usually solitary and occurs in young adults without a predilection site. The majority of these lesions are tender or painful, perhaps from contraction of myoepithelial cells and stimulation of the nerve fibers that are abundant in the capsules and occasionally in the parenchyma. Although it is usually a small (1- to 2-cm) intradermal or subcutaneous nodule, large tumors are also reported.[85,86] In rare instances multiple lesions are found.[87–89] They may be arranged in a linear[90] or a zoster-like distribution.[91] A histologic resemblance to dermal cylindroma is striking in some tumors,[92] and in fact both can coexist in the same patient.[93,94]

Histology

At low magnification this intradermal tumor resembles basal cell epithelioma or lymph node because of its densely packed, strongly basophilic cells (Fig. 2.35). However, it is usually deep seated and never shows connections with the epidermis or hair follicles. Dense, hyalinized collagen bundles often surround the tumor, which shows no palisading at the periphery. The basic construction of parenchyma is tubular (Fig. 2.35D). In a large tumor, however, such tubules are densely packed within a limited space and become so entangled that this basic structure is often obscured. On closer inspection, the outer layer of the tubules is composed of small basaloid cells with compact nuclei and the inner layer of larger, pale-staining cells (Figs. 2.35D and 2.36). Narrow and wide lumina, often resembling eccrine ducts and glandular spaces, are frequently found at the periphery of the parenchyma just inside the capsule. The stroma between interwoven cords of tumor cells is edematous and contains small blood vessels. Thus, when the stroma located between tumor tubules undergoes degeneration, it looks like a luminal space (Fig. 2.36). The hyalinized collagen capsules invaginate the tumor and send short septae into the peripheral parenchyma. The tips of these septae are branched and tapered; in thin sections (5 to 8 μ) of paraffin-embedded tissue, these branched tips are cut interrupted and therefore appear as hyalin droplets (Fig. 2.37). Normal or adenoid eccrine glands may lie close to the tumor (Figs. 2.35C, D and 2.36A), and in serial sections a connection can be demonstrated.

Histochemistry

Glycogen and eccrine-type enzymes (Table 1.3) are inconsistently demonstrated.[62,95] Nerve fibers surround the capsule and are demonstrable with acetylcholinesterase stain.[17] Small fibers are also present in the stroma within the tumor but are not as easily stained as in the capsule. The hyalinized capsule may be PAS positive and diastase resistant; the substance is therefore neutral mucopolysaccharide. The same substance is positive in the hyalin septae and in droplets within the tumor (Fig. 2.37).

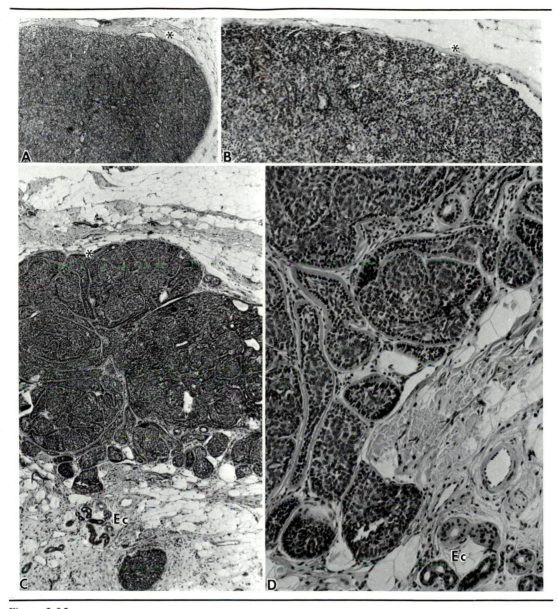

Figure 2.35
Eccrine spiradenoma. On low magnification an island of eccrine spiradenoma looks like a lymph node because of its small basophilic cells and its encapsulation (∗) by a thin rim of compressed collagen and hyalin membrane (A, B, and C). In a medium magnification the hyalin capsule or membrane is seen invaginating into the tumor parenchyma that accompanies the proliferation of tubular tumor strands (D). It can also be seen at this magnification that the tumor is essentially a continuous growth of glandular and ductal tubules that pile up and become entangled within a limited space (C, D). Normal eccrine glands in the vicinity (Ec in C and D) may be a part of the original structure from which the tumor developed. In D two types of cells are seen: small basophilic cells along the periphery of tubules and larger, pale cells toward the center. (A, × 22; B, × 52; C, × 130; D, × 163.)

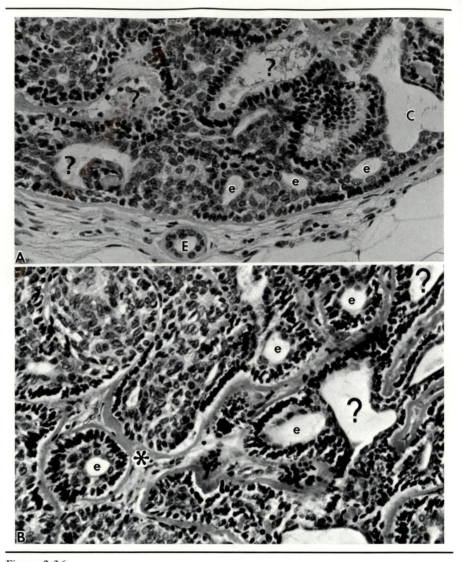

Figure 2.36
Eccrine spiradenoma. In A, three eccrine gland-like spaces (e) at the periphery are very similar to a true eccrine gland (E) that exists within the compressed collagen capsule. A large cystic space (C) may be the continuation of these spaces, whereas other debris-containing spaces (?) represent degenerated stroma. In B, typical eccrine gland-like structures (e) and large spaces created by degenerative stroma, that is, pseudolumina (?) are admixed. In A and B, peripherally located small, dense cells and centrally situated large, pale cells are recognized. Hyaline membranes surround individual tubules (*). (A and B, × 200.)

Electron Microscopy

Small basaloid cells are situated on the continuous, often thickened basal lamina and are connected to it with hemidesmosomes (Fig. 2.38). These correspond to the densely basophilic outer cells of the tubular structures seen on

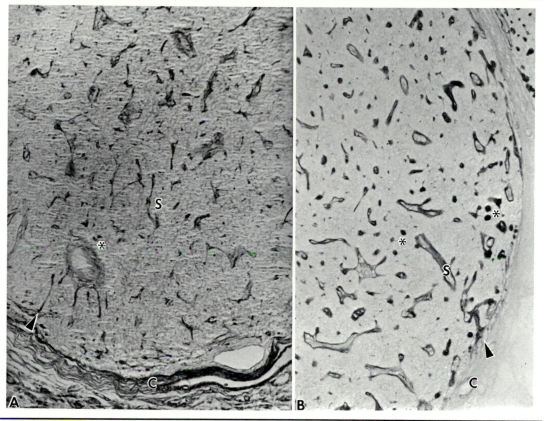

Figure 2.37
Eccrine spiradenoma. In A and B a PAS-positive, diastase-resistant capsule (C) continues into the tumor mass (arrowheads) and forms hyaline septae (S) and droplets (*). The latter can be seen when small branches are cross-sectioned. In B, the capsule is not stained. (A and B, × 130.)

light microscopy. Occasionally myoepithelial cells are wedged between the outer cells (Fig. 2.38). Inner cells are layered upon the basal cells; these are larger and have a higher cytoplasmic/nuclear ratio than the outer cells. Neither cell type shows any specific differentiation except for a small number of tonofilaments and poorly developed desmosomes. More differentiated structures such as ducts and glandular epithelia seem to develop from the inner cells (Fig. 2.39); they have therefore been named "indeterminate" cells.[95] Ductal epithelium lining the lumina often demonstrates numerous short villi and a periluminal band of tonofilaments (Fig. 2.39A); other lumina are lined with large cells having fewer tonofilaments and long, slender villi (Fig. 2.39B). The latter share general characteristics of secretory epithelium; if one assumes that this portion of the tumor is differentiating toward an eccrine secretory type, these large luminal cells with sparse, slender villi should correspond to clear (serous) cells of the normal eccrine gland. There are no tumor cells that contain mucous granules and could thus correspond to dark (mucous) cells. Some luminal cells discharge a part of their cytoplasm; a chain of small vesicles is

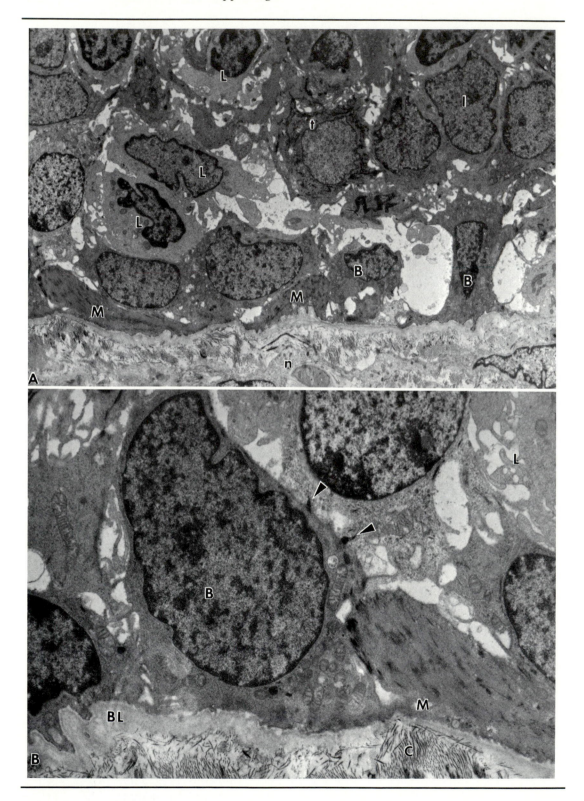

formed and segregates a portion of these cells as if they were engaged in apocrine (decapitation) secretion[95,96] (Fig. 2.39B). In some lumina the lining cells are composed of these three types (Fig. 2.39B). It is interesting to see decapitation secretion in eccrine spiradenoma, which by all criteria is an eccrine adenoma. Many tumor cells, particularly indeterminate cells, show centrioles whose extensions often form cilia or even flagella.[95]

The stroma contains unmyelinated axons within Schwann cells. Aggregated anchoring fibrils are admixed with thickened basal lamina-like materials surrounding the tumor islands. This feature will be illustrated with dermal cylindroma (Chapter 5; Figs. 5.15 and 5.17) because it is much more pronounced. The continuous coverage of basal cells of tubular cord with thickened basal lamina confirms that eccrine spiradenoma is essentially a tubular tumor of an eccrine dermal duct and a coiled secretory segment; as the tumor grows in a tightly bound space, these tubular ducts and coils become intertwined and form spirals. This feature is best visualized in less densely packed areas (Fig. 2.35C, D). The term *spiradenoma* was apparently used by Unna to designate coils of the secretory segment of the eccrine gland,[97] then was adopted by Kersting and Helwig.[98] The name seems to illustrate histologic features of the tumor. A large number of Langerhans' cells are seen migrating through the parenchyma (Fig. 2.38).

Malignant eccrine spiradenoma or *spiradenocarcinoma* is a rare tumor; only six cases have been reported.[99–102] It originates within a longstanding eccrine spiradenoma; therefore, one sees a transition from a still benign eccrine spiradenoma to a malignant tumor. Rapid enlargement with or without ulceration or cells spilling out of the capsule suggests peristromal invasion; disorganization of the two layer structures; mitosis, pleomorphism, and nuclear hyperchromasia are seen; and adenocarcinomatous pictures are well developed (Fig. 2.40). Tumor cells may show squamous metaplasia or spindle cell sarcoma-like transformation.

Eccrine Nevus

This tumor represents hyperplasia of normal mature eccrine secretory coils and may be associated with eccrine ducts (Fig. 2.41). Discharge from these secretory coils may cause hyperhidrosis, either in a localized area[103–105] (ephidrosis) or from a pore.[106] In *eccrine angiomatous nevus*, one or more nodules[107,108] or a solitary plaque[109] may be found. In addition to eccrine

Figure 2.38
Eccrine spiradenoma. In A *and* B *small basal (B) and myoepithelial cells (M) are situated along the periphery; these correspond to small basophilic cells seen in the light microscopy. Relatively large indeterminate cells (I) and histiocytes, mostly Langerhans cells (L), occupy the center of the tubule; these are large pale cells seen in the light microscopy. Some indeterminate cells contain more tonofilaments (t) than others. Poorly developed desmosomes (arrowheads in* B*) are infrequently present. Basal lamina (BL) is thickened and fine collagen fibers (C) abut upon it. n—nerve fiber. (*A*, × 3,000;* B*, × 7,000.)*

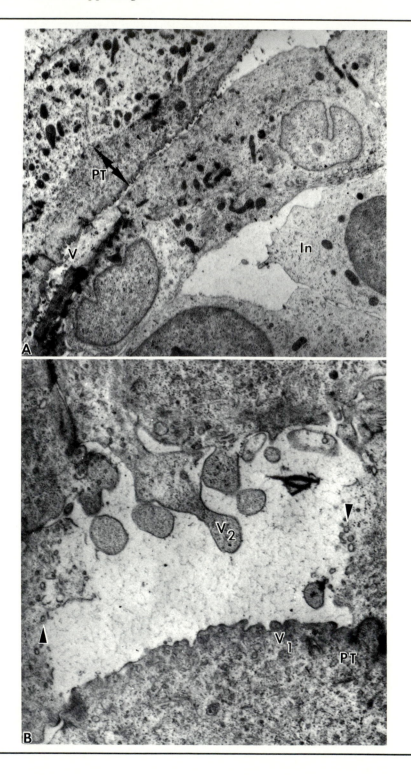

Figure 2.39
Eccrine spiradenoma. In A, ductal differentiation is seen: short but numerous villi (V) and periluminal dense layer (between arrows) of tonofilament aggregation (PT) are typical features of ductal epithelium. In B, one luminal cell shows ductal features such as short villi (V$_1$) and a periluminal tonofilament band (PT), while the one opposite to it shows the elongated, sparsely distributed villi (V$_2$) that are commonly seen in secretory epithelium. Two other luminal cells show a chain of small vesicles (arrowheads); the apical cytoplasm distal to these demarcation vesicles has already been segregated (decapitated) and disintegrated in the lumen. In—indeterminate cell. (A, × 5,750; B, × 14,500.)

hyperplasia, this variety has a vascular component. Sometimes the lesion is painful,[110] probably due to absence or inadequacy of ductal structures.

Histology

Secretory coils are increased in number and/or size. Usually, if multiple ducts are present, both the number and size may be increased,[103,104] whereas when a single duct is attached, only the size of the eccrine coil is augmented.[106] Figure 2.41 shows a case in which multiple ducts are attached to an eccrine nevus; the sizes of individual coils are, however, within the normal range of variation. In some cases the covering epidermis may show basaloid proliferation.[111] Small nerves may be admixed.[35] In *eccrine angiomatous hamartoma* or *nevus*, capillary as well as larger vessels are present, either surrounding the eccrine coils or admixed with them (Fig. 2.42).

Eccrine Duct Proliferation

Proliferation,[111] branching, squamous metaplasia, and cystic dilatation of an eccrine duct may occur alone or in association with other conditions such as keratoacanthoma.[112] Dilated ducts are often seen in the vicinity of various skin tumors and are probably due to compression and secondary obstruction. Weedon[35] states that squamous metaplasia (akin to sialometaplasia in the salivary gland) can be seen in ischemia, adjacent to ulcers, or following cryotherapy. Branched ductal structures as illustrated by Weedon[35] appear similar to his acrosyringeal nevus or the eccrine syringofibroadenoma described by Mascaro.[10]

Eccrine Adenoma

Adenomatous proliferation of the eccrine secretory segment may be seen as part of a papillary eccrine adenoma, representing adenomatous proliferation of the eccrine duct. It may also occur in association with various skin tumors.

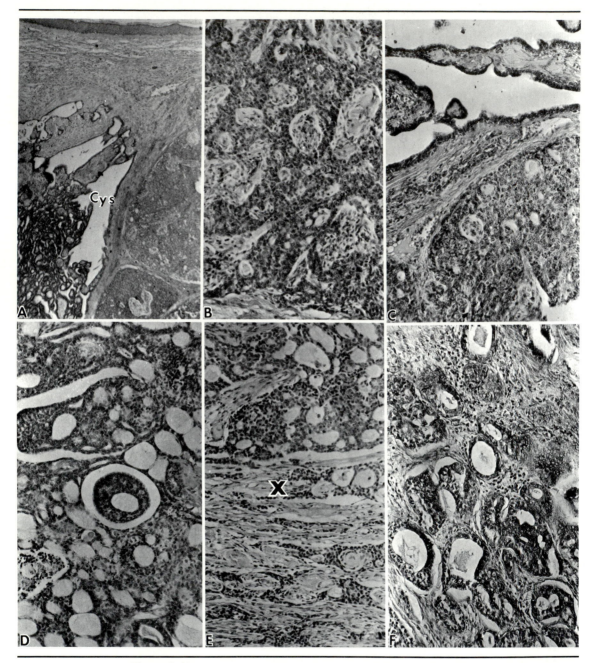

Figure 2.40

Malignant eccrine spiradenoma. In A, the eccrine spiradenoma-like, basophilic tumor has dilated peripheral cystic spaces (Cys) and more proliferative adenocarcinoma on the left, while more benign spiradenoma is still present on the right. Both areas are enlarged in C. In B, malignant cells are uniformly dense, and there is no distinction between peripheral small dense cells and central large pale cells. In D and F, adeno-carcinomatous features and cribriform vacuolation are evident. In E, an invasion of capsule and connective tissue (x) is seen. (A, × 33; B–F, × 163.)

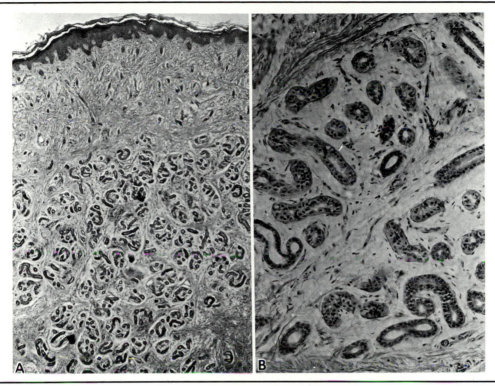

Figure 2.41
Eccrine nevus. Numerous groups of eccrine glands occupy the lower dermis. The up-
per dermis contains a number of ducts apparently connected to these glands (A). The
size and shape of these glands are almost normal except that some are rather elon-
gated and tubular and others have a slightly dilated lumina (B). (A, × 52; B, ×
163.)

Cutaneous Ciliated Cyst

This rare entity occurs predominantly in the lower extremities of young women[113–115]; however, Leonforte reported a lesion that occurred on the heel in a man.[116] This male case would refute the prevailing theory that the cyst represents Mullerian heterotopia because Fallopian tube epithelium requires a high level of estrogen for growth. The common location in the lower extremities,[114] particularly the sole of the foot,[134] negates an apocrine gland origin. The entity most likely represents a special type of eccrine ductal and/ or glandular differentiation. In fetal eccrine duct and in some eccrine lesions such as eccrine spiradenoma, cilia and flagella commonly develop.[96] Normal[115] or dilated[117] eccrine glands are found in the vicinity of the cyst.

Histology
The large, dilated cyst has a thin wall from which multiple projections extend into the cyst cavity (Fig. 2.43). Single or multiple layers of columnar epithe-

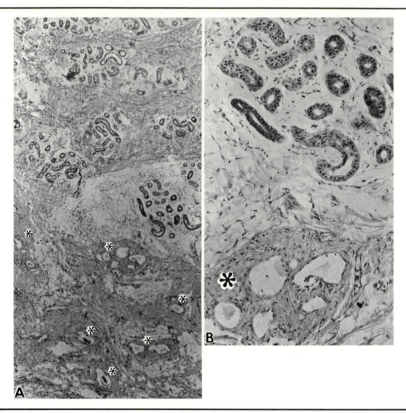

Figure 2.42
Eccrine angiomatous nevus. The lesion contains, in addition to a number of eccrine glands, many blood vessels (*) (A), some of which are thick-walled and have septate lumina (B). (A, × 33; B, × 163.)

lium line the wall. Most of these cells bear long, slender cilia, as can be confirmed by electron microscopy[116] (Fig. 2.44).

Bronchogenic Cyst

This is a rare congenital abnormality of the bronchial epithelium which by error ectopically develops in a subcutaneous location. It is usually noted shortly after birth as a small subcutaneous cyst with or without a draining sinus. Occasionally, however, older individuals develop the entity later in life. At low magnification (Fig. 2.45) the cyst resembles eccrine or apocrine hidrocystoma and is often diagnosed as such if one does not pay particular attention to the site of predilection: the lower anterior neck just above the sternal notch. Histologically, cystic spaces or sinuses are lined with ciliated epithelium (Fig. 2.45) and are often surrounded by inflammatory cell infiltrates.

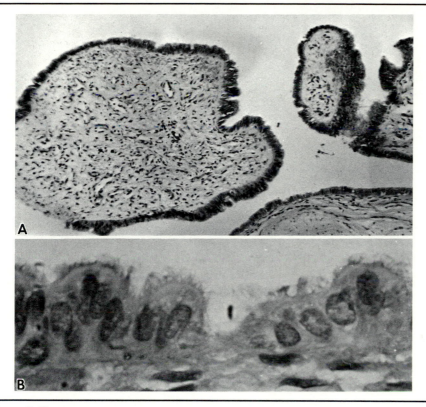

Figure 2.43
Cutaneous ciliated cyst. Papillary projections of the cyst wall extend into the cystic cavity. These projections are covered with a thin layer of columnar or cylindrical epithelium (A). *In* B, *the luminal surface of these columnar cells bears numerous hair-like structures (cilia).* (A, × 130; B, × 600.) (*Courtesy of José F. Leonforte, M.D.*)

Primary Eccrine Gland Carcinomas

In addition to the previously discussed instances in which malignancy occurs in a preexisting benign eccrine tumor (*e.g.,* malignant eccrine spiradenoma) or what are considered to be malignant counterparts of benign tumors (*e.g.,* malignant syringoacanthoma, porocarcinoma, etc.), several other histologic varieties of primary eccrine gland carcinomas have been recognized. These tumors are rare; in one series 35 cases were found among 450,000 consecutive skin biopsy specimens (0.007%).[32] Common sites of occurrence are the extremities and the head and neck region of elderly individuals.

The clinical appearance of eccrine gland carcinoma varies and therefore does not contribute to the diagnosis. Tissue diagnosis is relatively easy if one is informed of the histologic variations and can exclude the possibility of a metastatic adenocarcinoma. The most difficult task is to classify these tumors

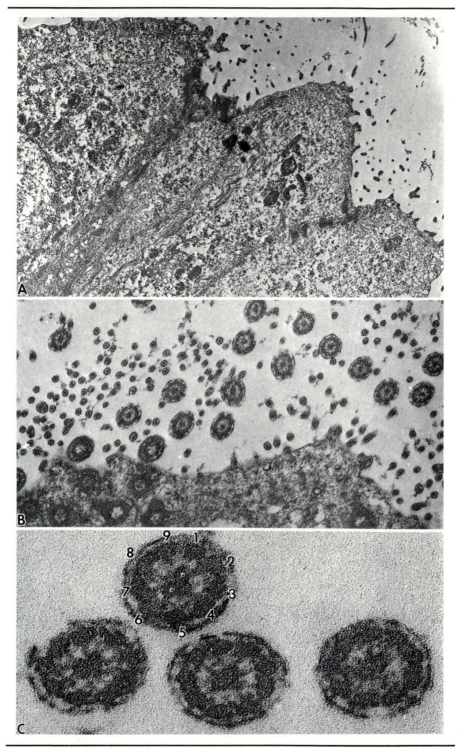

Figure 2.44
Cutaneous ciliated cyst. The luminal cells are covered with numerous villi on the luminal surface (A). On higher magnification cross-sections of these villi reveal an outer ring and central dots (B). In C, most of the cross-sectioned cilia show nine

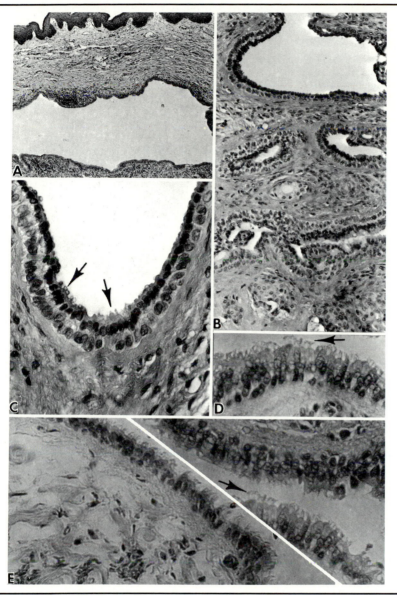

Figure 2.45
Bronchogenic cyst. In A, B, and C, dilated cystic spaces with irregularly projecting cystic walls closely resemble those of apocrine hidrocystoma (cf Fig. 5.3). On high magnification, however, what appeared to be decapitation secretion in C (arrows) is revealed to be a ciliated luminal border (arrows in D and E). (A, × 33; B, × 65; C, × 163; D and E, × 600.)

subunits in the outer ring and two dots in the center, that is, typical 9 + 2 cilial fibrils. (A, × 9,000; B, × 30,000; C, × 150,000.) (Courtesy of José F. Leonforte, M.D.)

into certain subtypes, although it is often of academic interest. Several authors have attempted to propose a uniformly acceptable classification of eccrine gland carcinomas; however, with the exception of a few well-defined varieties, their opinions have been challenged and refuted by new findings. Such difficulties seem to be related to three factors: (1) inadequate information because of the rarity of these tumors; (2) in view of the admixture of various components or subtypes in the same tumor, emphasis on one aspect or failure to examine each tumor completely in serial sectioning leads to a biased opinion; and (3) confusion over the cyst formation, whether the tumor space arises as a genuine glandular lumen or through pseudocyst formation by collagenolysis and mucin release or neogenesis of mucin by tumor cells.

Eccrine gland carcinomas are rare. In the world literature fewer than 200 cases have been reported, and the majority predate the modern era of histochemistry, electron microscopy, and immunohistochemistry. Except for a few subtypes in which one structural pattern predominates (*i.e.,* syringoid, clear cell, and mucinous eccrine carcinomas), the majority of "eccrine adenocarcinomas" of the classic type are made up of several often entirely different components. The degree of malignancy as judged from structural disorganization (more solid-cellular than glandular), cellular atypia (giant cells, bizarre nuclei), hyperchromatic nuclei, and mitotic activity also varies from one part of the tumor to another. (Three examples of this type are given in Figs. 2.50–2.52.) Composite pictures in each plate were taken from various parts of the same lesion; considerable variation in architecture and degree of malignancy is evident. These tumors are most likely polyclonal in origin with each clone achieving its own structural goal.

The third difficulty in classifying these lesions results from lack of definition of the "cyst" or lack of knowledge about its histogenesis. Some spaces formed within the tumor mass or parenchyma are produced by collagen degeneration and/or mucin production, the same mechanism which in basal cell epithelioma produces retraction spaces. It is due to collagenase digestion of stromal collagen and mucin release from degenerated collagen molecules. True glandular or ductal spaces or cysts surrounded by secretory or ductal epithelium certainly exist among these tumor islands. However, most of the large, irregularly shaped spaces within big tumor islands (see Fig. 2.53D) and cribriform microcysts (see Fig. 2.52E) are secondary to collagenolytic activity. Fragments of collagen, fibroblasts, and/or erythrocytes are often found in these lumina. Electron microscopy does not detect either secretory or ductal luminal cells. In the discussion that follows, the well-defined and recognized group of eccrine carcinomas is addressed first; the eccrine adenocarcinoma group is then analyzed.

Syringoid Eccrine Carcinoma

This tumor is usually a solitary one and occurs in the extremities and the head and face region of elderly individuals.[32] Infiltrated plaque-like lesions of the scalp may show alopecia.[32]

Histology

The tumor may be connected to the epidermis with a dilated ductal space open to the surface (Fig. 2.46); the area is acanthotic or papillary and may suggest syringocystadenoma papilliferum (Fig. 2.46). Tubular adenoid structures resemble syringoma, but mitosis, irregular cell size, and the nuclear chro-

Figure 2.46
Syringoid eccrine carcinoma. In A, papillary and verrucous (v) epidermis invaginates (arrowhead) into an adenocystic lesion. In B, tubulocystic structures predominate and connect both with each other (**) and with a keratin cyst (*). Small cystic lesions attached to an epithelial cord resemble the tadpole picture of typical syringoma (s). In C, one of the tubuloductal structures (arrow) is connected to the epidermis (E). (A, × 65; B, × 52; C, × 200.)

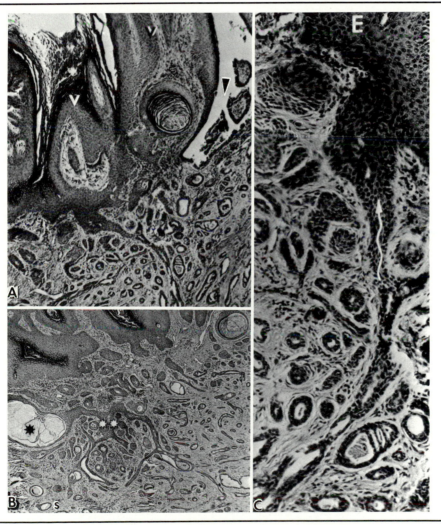

matin pattern suggest malignancy (Fig. 2.47). The stroma may be vascular or fibrotic, in some cases even chondroid. The full thickness of the dermis, and in some cases the subcutaneous fat layer, is involved.

Electron Microscopy

As in syringoma (Fig. 2.25), the epithelial lining of the adenocystic lumina may contain keratinized or ductal cells.[117] In addition, secretory-type cells (Fig. 2.48) may be present.

Figure 2.47
Syringoid (adenoid cystic) eccrine carcinoma. In A and B large cystic space (C) and adenoid lesions (A) are present in these areas of the same tumor shown in Fig. 2.46. In C, atypia, hyperchromasia, and papillary growth (*) are shown. (A and B, × 130; C, × 163.)

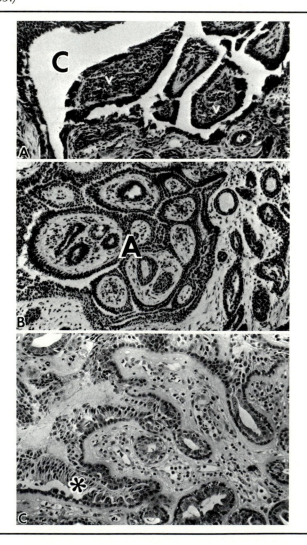

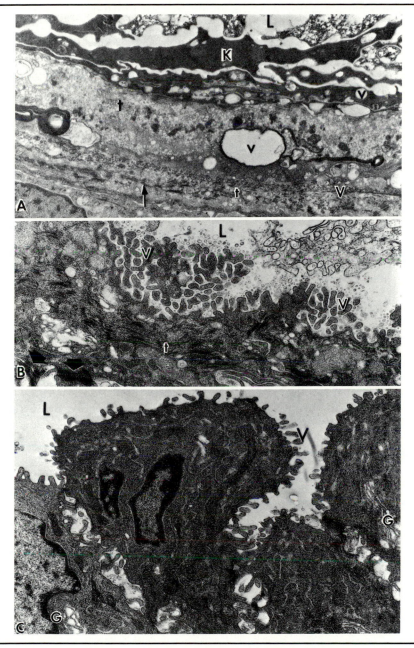

Figure 2.48
*Syringoid eccrine carcinoma. In A, the lumen (L) is lined with keratinized cells (K).
Nonkeratinized wall cells contain many vacuoles (V). Tonofilament bundles (t) and
desmosomes (arrow) are present. In B, ductal differentiation of luminal cells is seen:
short but numerous villi (V) project into the lumen and the periluminal tonofilament
band (t) is formed. Arrows indicate desmosomal connections. In C, the large plump
cells are secretory-type cells with Golgi cisterns (G) and long but sparsely populated
villi (V) that project into the lumen (L). (A, × 8,000; B, × 12,000; C, × 12,000.)*

Eccrine Epithelioma or Eccrine Differentiation of Basal Cell Epithelioma

Eccrine epithelioma or eccrine differentiation of basal cell epithelioma was first described by Freeman and Winkelmann[118] and then by Sanchez and Winkelmann.[119] Weedon[54] identified a spectrum of basal cell epitheliomas that exhibited prominent differentiation toward eccrine gland. Histologically, in addition to branching tubular structures, solid clumps of basaloid cells and masses with an adenoid pattern are seen (Fig. 2.49). Eccrine epitheliomas are rarely connected with the overlying epidermis. They are locally destructive but show no tendency for local lymph node involvement or distant metastasis.[118,119]

Mucinous Eccrine Carcinoma

This tumor is an uncommon variety of eccrine carcinoma; fewer than 40 cases have been reported[120–127] since Mendoza and Helwig[128] described the first patient in 1971. Eyelid lesions, present in 23 of the 40 cases, are somewhat frequently reported in the ophthalmologic literature.[120–123] The tumor is usually a single nodule, and widespread metastasis is rare.[125] Histologic study reveals small solid nests or adenoid structures that are made up of small basaloid cells (Fig. 2.50). Tumor nests characteristically float in the pools of mucinous stroma, which is alcian blue positive.[32] Mucinous pools may coalesce or sclerotic collagen septae may separate them. The tumor nests or tubular structures are populated with basaloid cells. However, upon close observation, many features of malignancy can be detected; for example, cellular atypia, hyperchromatic nuclei, and occasional mitotic figures (Fig. 2.50).

Clear Cell Eccrine Carcinoma

This rare variety has been classified under various names, including malignant clear cell hidradenoma,[129] clear cell hidradenocarcinoma,[130,131] and malignant clear cell acrospiroma.[132] The tumor is solitary and commonly occurs in the face and head region or the extremities, particularly on the hands and feet. A case of congenital tumor on the cheek has also been reported by Hernandez-Perez and Cruz.[131] Extensive metastasis is common.

Histology

This variety is often difficult to differentiate from benign clear cell hidradenoma or acrospiroma because cellular pleomorphism is not prominent on light and electron microscopy.[132] Even metastatic lesions may appear benign.[131] Eccrine-type enzymes and glycogen are abundant,[132] suggesting advanced cellular differentiation. A few mitotic figures and an irregular periphery with invasive features may suggest the malignant nature of the lesion (Fig. 2.51). Solid, adenoid, and tubulocystic portions may be recognized in the same tumor; in all these structural variations the clear cells and cellular atypia are the common denominator.[133,134,135] Without large, glycogen-rich clear cells,

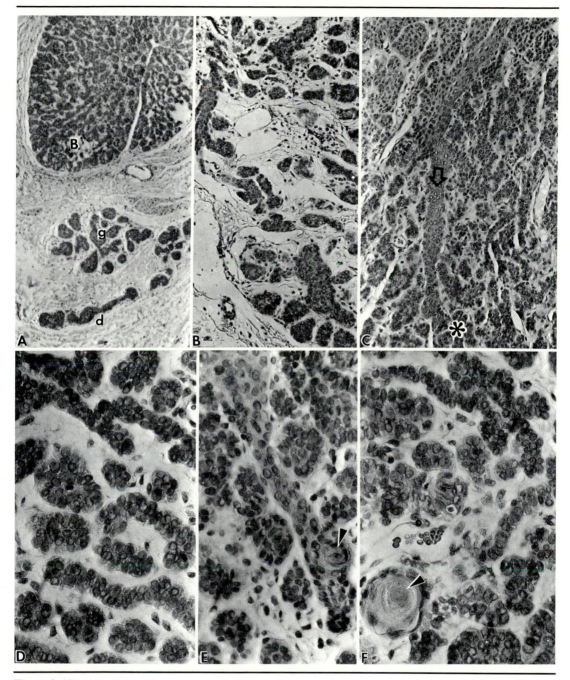

Figure 2.49
*Eccrine epithelioma. In A, the main lesion of basal cell epithelioma (B) is rather
thready or tubular. Eccrine sweat gland-like (g) and eccrine duct-like (d) structures
underlie the main mass. In B and D, tubular and rosette-form structures are magnified. In C, a ductal structure (arrow) extends from the epidermis; its tip forms rosettes (*). In E and F, a cross-section of ductal lumen formation is seen
(arrowheads). (A, × 35; B and C, × 65; D–F, × 163.)*

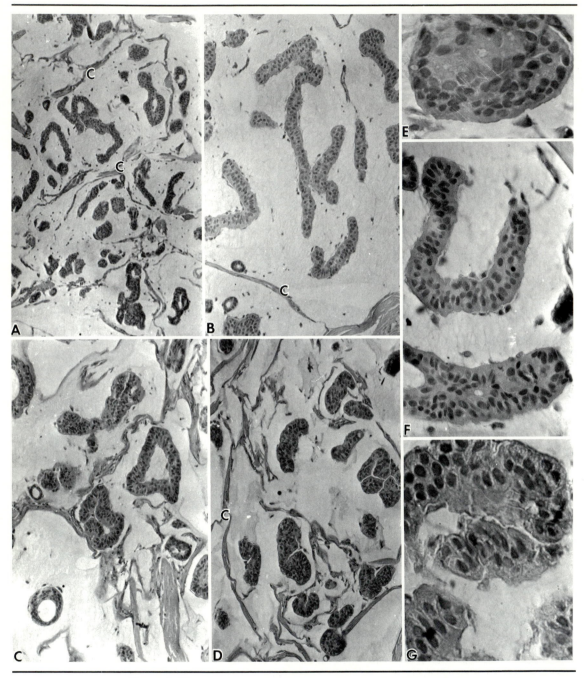

Figure 2.50
Mucinous eccrine carcinoma. Tubular and microcystic structures resemble eccrine glands (A, B, and C) except that these are irregular in size and shape, and lumen formation is often absent in tubular structures (B) and epithelial masses (D). Cellular atypia is evident (E, F, and G). The most striking features are the pools of mucin that embed these tumors. Thin septae of collagenous tissue (C in A, B, and D) separate individual mucinous pools. (A–D, × 130; E–G, × 520.)

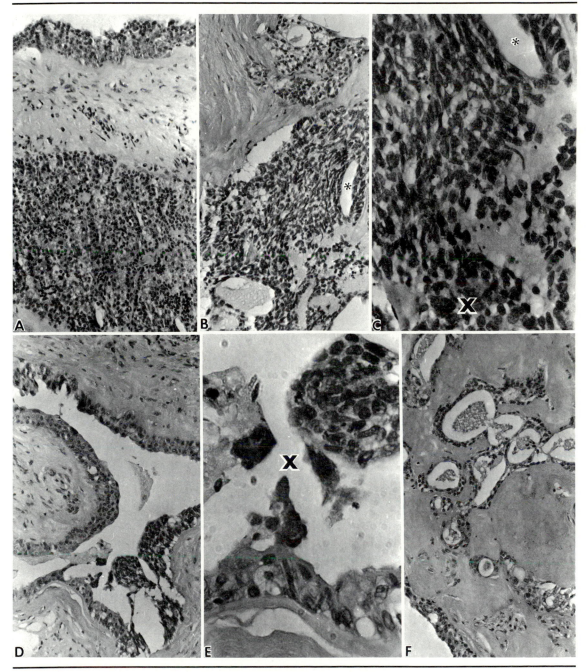

Figure 2.51
*Clear cell eccrine carcinoma. In A a large proportion of tumor cells in solid areas
are clear cells, otherwise these pictures are similar to malignant eccrine spiradenoma
(cf Fig. 2.40). In B, and C, glandular lumen formation (*) is seen. In D, there is a
large cystic space, and in f, syringoid structures are produced. Cellular atypia (x) is
evident in C and E. Stroma is fibrotic or even chondroid in B and F. All pictures
were taken from the same specimen. (A, B, and F, × 65; D, × 130; C and E, × 520.)*

some portions of clear cell eccrine carcinoma can easily be mistaken for malignant eccrine spiradenoma (Fig. 2.51A, B, C), syringocystadenoma papilliferum (Fig. 2.51D), chondroid syringoma (Fig. 2.51F), and other types of
eccrine carcinomas such as aggressive digital papillary adenocarcinoma.

Eccrine Adenocarcinoma

Eccrine adenocarcinoma, the classic type of eccrine gland carcinoma, is a
rapidly growing, highly metastatic tumor. El-Domeiri et al. reported five-year
follow-up of 68 cases; 29 patients had regional lymph node metastasis and
26 showed visceral metastases.[133]

Histology

The basic architecture is adenocystic (Fig. 2.52A, D). However, many variations exist: solid-cellular (Fig. 2.52B), tubular (Fig. 2.52C), basalioma-like,
squamoid, among others. These subtypes may be seen within the same tumor.
When all or parts of a tumor show the solid-cellular pattern, the inflammatory
response is usually severe, and it is often difficult to distinguish tumor cells
from inflammatory infiltrates (Fig. 2.52B). Eccrine-type enzymes and glycogen
are present in the tumor cells, particularly in the clear cells found in glandular
structures (Fig. 2.52E). PAS stain is therefore very useful for differentiating a
highly invasive, cellular variety from metastatic adenocarcinoma. Electron microscopy may demonstrate intracellular multiple cavity formation, which
mimics embryonic production of the eccrine acrosyringeal duct (Fig. 2.52F).
Although this mode of ductal space formation occasionally occurs with adenocarcinomas of the gastrointestinal tract, its frequency in eccrine adenocarcinoma is a valuable aid in differential diagnosis.

Adenoid Cystic Eccrine Carcinoma

This variety, first described by Boggio[134] in 1975, consists of a large epithelial
island with adenoid or cribriform features (Fig. 2.53A–J). Such a pattern may

Figure 2.52
*Eccrine adenocarcinoma, classic type. In A, atypical wall cells protrude into large
glandular lumina (arrowheads). Some tumor cells seem to be shed into the luminal
spaces. In B, the solid-cellular (S) and glandular portions (G) are mixed; the latter
has many clear or vacuolated cells. In C, the tubular or basalioma-like portions consist of two parallel rows of basaloid cells and, in some centers (*), squamous metaplasia. In D, atypical glandular differentiation and nuclear atypia (arrowheads) are
evident. In E, PAS stain demonstrates glycogen in cavity-forming tumor islands. In
F, an electron micrograph shows intracellular, multiple (1, 2, 3) cavity formation.
The wall of each cavity is typically ductal with differentiation of numerous short villi
(V). All pictures were taken from the same lesion. (A, × 100; B and C, × 130; D
and E, × 520; F, × 10,000.)*

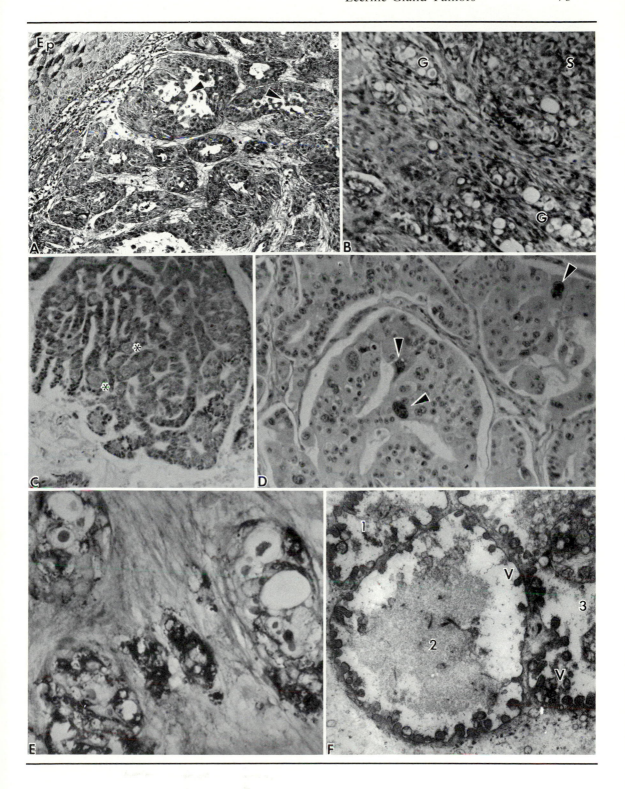

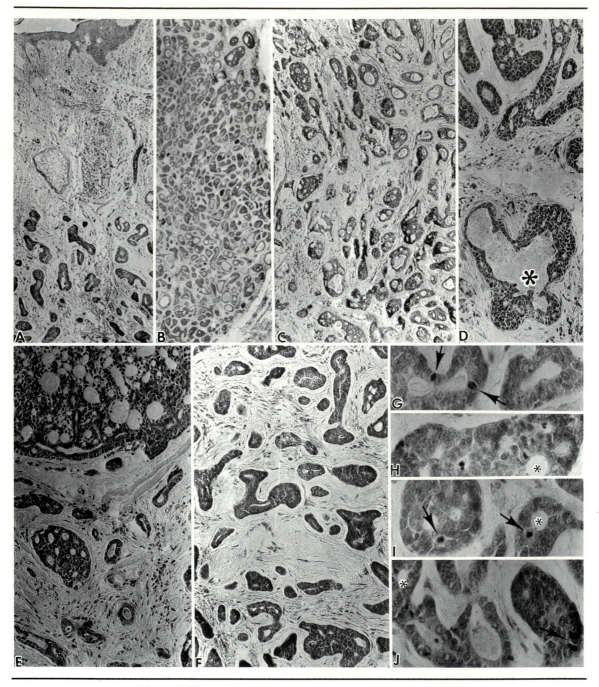

Figure 2.53
*Adenoid cystic eccrine carcinoma, classic type. A variety of subtypes are admixed in
this tumor. In A, B, and C, a relatively well-differentiated or* syringoid *pattern is
seen.* Adenoid cystic (D) *or* cribriform (E) *patterns are also obvious although in D
the cyst-like spaces are mostly pseudocysts (*). In F, a basalioma-like pattern with
clear space formation surrounding each tumor island is observed; this picture may
represent* eccrine epithelioma *(cf Fig. 2.49). In G, H, I, and J, glandular lumen formation (*) is seen. Despite well-formed structural maturity mitotic figures are frequent (arrow) in G–J. (A and C, × 33; B, × 22; D–F, × 130; G–J, × 153.)*

mimic adenoid basal cell epithelioma. The tumor may show mucinous degeneration of stroma surrounded by parenchyma; it may appear as if mucin is secreted by the tumor cells (Fig. 2.53D).[134] The stroma surrounding small tubular structures or epithelial islands may also undergo mucinous degeneration (Fig. 2.53F). Because this pattern is often seen in basal cell epithelioma, it may be interpreted as eccrine differentiation of basal cell epithelioma.[119] Adenocystic eccrine carcinomas, like basal cell epitheliomas, may produce a cytokine that stimulates fibroblasts in the stroma to manufacture excessive collagenase.[136] The adenoid cystic variety may be related in this respect to mucinous eccrine carcinoma, which has also been called adenocystic eccrine carcinoma.[118,135] The true gland formation with differentiation of luminal epithelium should be clearly separated from pseudogland formation due to col-

Figure 2.54
Microcystic eccrine carcinoma. The dilated cystic spaces on the right are lined with cuboidal eccrine-type epithelium. Two islands on the left are more solidly epithelial than cystic. (× 225.)

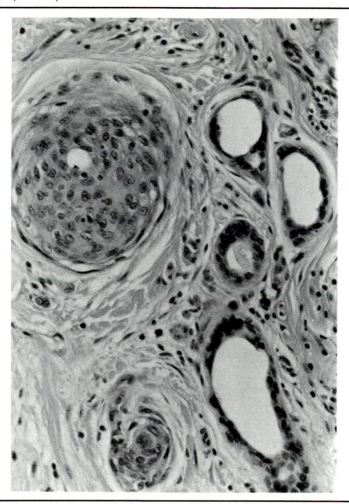

lagenolysis of the stroma. In most cases, adenocystic spaces in mucinous eccrine carcinoma are formed by collagenolysis or the accumulation of mucin. In adenoid cystic eccrine carcinoma, cribriform structures and large cystic spaces in the center of epithelial islands (as depicted in Fig. 2.53E and D respectively) are formed by collagenolytic action, not by true gland formation.

Microcystic Eccrine Carcinoma

Originally described by Goldstein et al.[137] in 1982 as microcystic adnexal carcinoma, this lesion most commonly occurs over the upper lip and cheeks

Figure 2.55
Microcystic eccrine carcinoma. This lesion is very similar to syringoma or syringoid eccrine carcinoma in that these cystic spaces contain eosinophilic substances (*) that consist of keratin and lysosomal debris, and they have frequent attachment of tadpole tail-like epithelial cords (arrowheads). Independent epithelial cords (e) are also noticed. Sclerotic stroma is also similar to that commonly seen in syringoma. (× 225.)

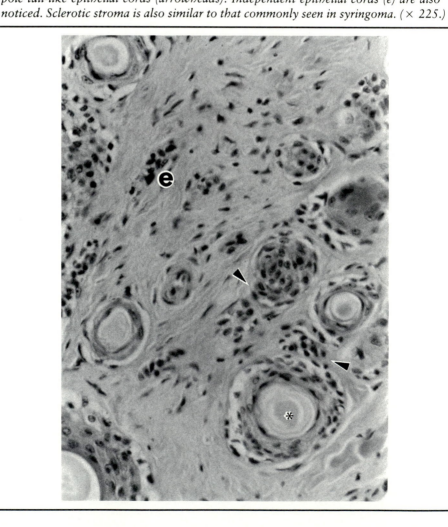

as a nodular growth with deep dermal infiltration.[138] Histologically, a combination of small solid nests and thin strands of basaloid cells, keratin cysts, and duct-like structures is embedded in a hyalinized fibrous stroma[139] (Figs. 2.54 and 2.55). The growth extends into subcutaneous fat and may show areas of perivascular and perineural involvement. There is a tendency for local recurrence following surgical excision. A 30-year follow-up in a single case suggested that this is a slow-growing neoplasm.[140]

REFERENCES

1. Pinkus H, Rogin J, Goldman P. Eccrine poroma. Arch Dermatol 1956;74:511–521.
2. Hyman AB, Brownstein MH. Eccrine poroma. An analysis of 45 new cases. Dermatologica 1969;138:29–38.
3. Okun MR, Ansell HB. Eccrine poroma. Arch Dermatol 1963;88:561–566.
4. Penneys NS, Ackerman AB, Indgin SN, et al. Eccrine poroma. Br J Dermatol 1970;82:613–615.
5. Winkelmann RK, Wolff K. Solid-cystic hidradenoma of the skin: clinical and histologic study. Arch Dermatol 1968;97:651–661.
6. Johnson BL Jr, Helwig EB. Eccrine acrospiroma: a clinicopathologic study. Cancer 1969;23:651–657.
7. Winkelmann RK, McLeod WA. The dermal duct tumor. Arch Dermatol 1966;94:50–55.
8. Goldner R. Eccrine poromatosis. Arch Dermatol 1970;101:606–608.
9. Wilkinson RD, Schopflocher P, Rozenfeld M. Hidrotic ectodermal dysplasia with diffuse eccrine poromatosis. Arch Dermatol 1977;113:472–476.
10. Mascaro JM. Considerations sur les tumeurs fibro-epitheliales. Le syringofibroadenome eccrine. Ann Derm Syph 1963;90:146–153.
11. Olmos L. Syringofibroadenoma ecrino de Mascaro. Acta Dermosifilogr 1980;71:73–76.
12. Civatte J, Jeanmougin M, Barrandon Y, Jimenez de Franch. Siringo-fibroadenoma ecrino de Mascaro. Discusion de un Caso. Med Cut I.L.A. 1981;9:193–196.
13. Mehregan A, Marufi M, Medenica M. Eccrine syringofibroadenoma (Mascaro). Report of two cases. J Am Acad Dermatol 1985;13:433–436.
14. Pinkus H. Epithelial and fibroepithelial tumors. Arch Dermatol 1965;91:24–37.
15. Weedon D, Lewis J. Acrosyringeal nevus. J Cutan Pathol 1977;4:166–168.
16. Weedon D: Personal communication.
17. Ogino A. Linear eccrine poroma. Arch Dermatol 1976;112:841–844.
18. Blanchard L, Hodge SJ, Owen LG. Linear eccrine nevus with comedones. Arch Dermatol 1981;117:357–359.
19. Abell E, Read SI. Porokeratotic eccrine ostial and dermal duct naevus. Br J Dermatol 1980;103:435–441.
20. Marsden RA, Fleming K, Dawber RPR: Comedo naevus of the palm—A sweat duct naevus. Br J Dermatol 1979;101:717–722.
21. Coskey RJ, Mehregan AH, Hashimoto K. Porokeratotic eccrine duct and hair follicle nevus. J Am Acad Dermatol 1982;6:940–943.
22. Shaw JJ, White CR. Porokeratosis plantaris palmaris et disseminata. J Am Acad Dermatol 1984;11:454–460.
23. Rahbari H. Syringoacanthoma. Acanthotic lesion of the acrosyringium. Arch Dermatol 1984;120:751–756.

24. Smith JLS, Coburn JG. Hidroacanthoma simplex: Assessment of selected group of intraepidermal basal cell epitheliomata and of their malignant homologues. Br J Dermatol 1956;68:400–418.
25. Mehregan AH, Levson D. Hidroacanthoma simplex: A report of two cases. Arch Dermatol 1969;100:303–305.
26. Borst M. Ueber die Möglichkeit einer ausgedehnten intraepidermalen verbreitung des hautkrebses. Verh Dtsch Ges Pathol 1904;7:118–123.
27. Mehregan AH, Pinkus H. Intraepidermal epithelioma: A critical study. Cancer 1964;17:609–636.
28. Pinkus H, Mehregan AH. Epidermotropic eccrine carcinoma. Arch Dermatol 1963;88:597–606.
29. Mishima Y, Morioka S. Oncogenic differentiation of the intraepidermal sweat duct: Eccrine poroma, poroepithelioma and porocarcinoma. Dermatologica 1969;138:238–250.
30. Bardach H. Hidroacanthoma simplex with in situ porocarcinoma. J Cutan Pathol 1978;5:236–248.
31. Gschnait F, Horn F, Lindlbauer R, et al. Eccrine porocarcinoma. J Cutan Pathol 1980;7:349–353.
32. Mehregan AH, Hashimoto K, Rahbari H: Eccrine adenocarcinoma: A clinico-pathologic study of 35 cases. Arch Dermatol 1983;9:104–114.
33. Johnson BL, Helwig EB. Eccrine acrospiroma: A clinicopathologic study. Cancer 1969;23:641–657.
34. Helwig EB. Eccrine acrospiroma. J Cutan Pathol 1984;11:415–420.
35. Weedon D. Eccrine tumors: A selective review. J Cutan Pathol 1984;11:421–436.
36. Hashimoto K, DiBella RJ, Lever WF. Clear cell hidradenoma: Histological, histochemical, and electron microscopic studies. Arch Dermatol 1967;96:18–38.
37. Winkelmann RK, Wolf K. Histochemistry of hidradenoma and eccrine spiradenoma. J Invest Dermatol 1967;49:173–180.
38. Hashimoto K, Gross BG, Lever WF. Syringoma: Histochemical and electron microscopic studies. J Invest Dermatol 1966;46:150–166.
39. Hashimoto K, DiBella RJ, Borsuk GM. Eruptive hidradenoma and syringoma. Arch Dermatol 1967;96:500–519.
40. Jacquet L, Darier J. Hidradenomes éruptifs: I. Epitheliomes adenoides des glandes sudoripares. Ann Derm Syph 1887;8:317–323.
41. Yesudian P, Thambiah A. Familial syringoma. Dermatologica 1975;150:32–35.
42. Thomas J, Majmudar B, Gorelkin L. Syringoma localized to the vulva. Arch Dermatol 1979;115:95–96.
43. Zalla JA, Perry HO. An unusual case of syringoma. Arch Dermatol 1971;103:215–217.
44. Hughes PSH, Apisarnthanarax P. Acral syringoma. Arch Dermatol 1977;113:1435–1436.
45. Yung CW, Soltani K, Bernstein JE, et al. Unilateral linear nevoidal syringoma. J Am Acad Dermatol 1981;4:412–416.
46. Shelley WB, Wood MG. Occult syringomas of scalp associated with progressive hair loss. Arch Dermatol 1980;116:843–844.
47. Trozak DJ, Wood C. Occult eccrine sweat duct hamartoma and cicatricial scalp alopecia. Cutis 1984;34:475–477.
48. Dupré A, Bonafé JL, Christol B: Syringomas as a causative factor for cicatricial alopecia. Arch Dermatol 1981;117:315.
49. Holden CA, MacDonald DM. Syringomata: A bathing trunk distribution. Clin Exp Dermatol 1981;6:555–559.

50. Wilms NA, Douglass MC. An unusual case of preponderantly right-sided syringomas. Arch Dermatol 1981;117:308.

51. van der Broek H, Lundquist CD. Syringomas of the upper extremities with onset in the sixth decade. J Am Acad Dermatol 1982;6:534–536.

52. Butterworth T, Strean LP, Beerman H, Wood MG. Syringoma and mongolism. Arch Dermatol 1964;90:483–487.

53. Urban CD, Cannon JR, Cole RD. Eruptive syringomas in Down's syndrome. Arch Dermatol 1981;117:374–375.

54. Dupré A, Bonafé JL: Syrigomes, mongolisme, maladie de marfan et syndrome d'Ehlers–Danlos. Ann Dermatol Venereol 1977;104:224–230.

55. Hashimoto K, Gross BG, Lever WF. The ultrastructure of the skin of human embryos. I. The intraepidermal eccrine sweat duct. J Invest Dermatol 1965; 45:139–151.

56. Headington JT, Koski J, Murphy PJ. Clear cell glycogenosis in multiple syringomas: Description and enzyme histochemistry. Arch Dermatol 1972;106:353–356.

57. Kitamura K, Muraki R, Tamura N. Clear cell syringoma. Cutis 1983;32:169–172.

58. Mishima Y. Eccrine-centered nevus. Arch Dermatol 1973;107:59–61.

59. Schellander F, Marks R, Wilson Jones E. Basal cell hamartoma and cellular naevus: An unusual combined malformation. Br J Dermatol 1974;90:413–419.

60. Seifert HW. [Association of disseminated syringoma and mast cells clinically resembling urticaria pigmentosa]. Z Hautkr 1981;56:303–306.

61. Penneys NS. Immunohistochemistry of adnexal neoplasms. J Cutan Pathol 1984;11:357–364.

62. Hashimoto K, Lever WF. Histogenesis of some appendage tumors on the basis of histochemical and electron microscopic findings. Arch Dermatol 1969;100:356–369.

63. Mills SE. Mixed tumor of the skin: A model of divergent differentiation. J Cutan Pathol 1984;11:382–386.

64. Harrist TJ, Aretz TH, Mihm MC Jr, et al. Cutaneous malignant mixed tumor. Arch Dermatol 1981;117:719–724.

65. Botha JBC, Kahn LB. Aggressive chondroid syringoma. Arch Dermatol 1984;114:954–955.

66. Hilton JMN, Blackwell JB. Metastasizing chondroid syringoma. J Pathol 1973;109:167–170.

67. Matz LR, McCully DJ, Stokes BAR. Metastasizing chondroid syringoma: Case report. Pathology 1969;1:77–81.

68. Mills SE, Cooper PH. An ultrastructural study of cartilaginous zones and surrounding epithelium in mixed tumors of salivary glands and skin. Lab Invest 1981;44:6–12.

69. Johns ME, Mills SE, Thompson KK. Colony forming assay of human salivary gland tumors: Applications for chemosensitivity and histogenetic studies. Arch Otolaryngol 1981;109:709–714.

70. Varela-Duran J, Diaz-Flores L, Varella-Nunez R. Ultrastructure of chondroid syringoma. Cancer 1979;44:148–156.

71. Headington JT. Mixed tumors of the skin: Eccrine and apocrine types. Arch Dermatol 1961;84:989–996.

72. Hernandez FJ. Mixed tumors of the skin of the salivary type: A light and electron microscopic study. J Invest Dermatol 1976;66:49–52.

73. Hirsch P, Helwig EB. Chondroid syringoma. Arch Dermatol 1961;84:835–847.

74. Smith JD, Chernosky ME. Hidrocystomas. Arch Dermatol 1973;108:676–679.

75. Cordero AA, Montes LF. Eccrine hidrocystoma. J Cutan Pathol 1976;3:292–293.

76. Ebner H, Erlach E. Ekkrine Hidrozystome. Dermatol Monatsschr 1975;161:739–744.

77. Hassan MO, Khan MA. Ultrastructure of eccrine cystadenoma. Arch Dermatol 1979;115:1217–1221.

78. Rulon DB, Helwig EB. Papillary eccrine adenoma. Arch Dermatol 1977;113:596–598.

79. Elpern DJ, Farmer ER. Papillary eccrine adenoma. Arch Dermatol 1978;114:1241.

80. Sina B, Dilaimy M, Kallayee D. Papillary eccrine adenoma. Arch Dermatol 1980;116:719–720.

81. White SW, Rodman OG. Papillary eccrine adenoma. J Natl Med Assoc 1982;74:573–576.

82. Umbert P, Winkelmann RK. Tubular apocrine adenoma. J Cutan Pathol 1976;3:75–87.

83. Graham JH. Aggressive digital papillary adenoma. In: Proceedings of the XIV International Congress, International Academy of Pathology Meeting, Sydney, Australia, 1982.

84. Graham JH. Aggressive digital papillary adenoma and adenocarcinoma. Presented at the American Dermatological Association, One Hundred Fifth Annual Meeting, San Diego, Calif. 1985.

85. Lauret P, Boullie MC, Thomine E, Stewart WW. Giant eccrine spiradenoma. Ann Dermatol Vénéreol 1977;104:485–487.

86. Martin-Pascual A, Morán M, Bravo J, Armijo J. Giant eccrine spiradenoma. Actas Dermosifiliogr 1980;7:233–236.

87. Maia M, Proenca NG, Müller H. Espiradenomas ecrines multiplos. A proposito de dois casos em irmas. Med Cutan Iber Lat Am 1977;5:339–345.

88. Everall J, Dowd P. Multiple eccrine spiradenomata. Br J Dermatol 1979;101 (Suppl 17):33–34.

89. Bazex A, Dupré A, Cristol B, Cantala P. Spiradénomes eccrines multiples. Bull Soc Fr Dermatol Syphiligr 1971;78:73–74.

90. Tsur H, Lipskier E, Fisher BK. Multiple linear spiradenomas. Plast Reconstr Surg 1981;68:100–102.

91. Shelly WB, Wood MG. A zosteriform network of spiradenomas. J Am Acad Dermatol 1981;2:59–61.

92. Brownstein MH, Shapiro L. The sweat gland adenomas. Int J Dermatol 1975;14:397–411.

93. Goette DK, McConnell MA, Fowler VR. Cylindromas and eccrine spiradenoma coexistent in the same lesion. Arch Dermatol 1982;118:273–274.

94. Gerber JE, Descalzi ME. Eccrine spiradenoma and dermal cylindroma. J Cutan Pathol 1983;10:73–78.

95. Hashimoto K, Gross BG, Nelson RG, et al. Eccrine spiradenoma. Histochemical and electron microscopic studies. J Invest Dermatol 1966;46:347–365.

96. Hashimoto K. Ultrastructure of human apocrine glands. In: Jarrett A, ed. Physiology and pathophysiology of the skin. London: Academic Press, 5:1575–1596.

97. Unna PG. The histopathology of diseases of the skin. Walker, N, trans. Edinburgh: WF Clay, 1896;803–814.

98. Kersting DW, Helwig EB. Eccrine spiradenoma. Arch Dermatol 1956;73:199–227.

99. Dabska M. Malignant transformation of eccrine spiradenoma. Pol Med J 1972;11:388–396.

100. Evans HL, Su WPD, Smith JL, et al. Carcinoma arising in eccrine spiradenoma. Cancer 1979;43:1881–1884.

101. Cooper PH, Frierson HF Jr, Morrison G. Malignant transformation of eccrine spiradenoma. Arch Dermatol 1985;121:1445–1448.

102. Mambo NC. Eccrine spiradenoma: Clinical and pathologic study of 49 tumors. J Cutan Pathol 1983;10:312–320.

103. Arnold HL: Nevus seborrheicus et sudoriferus. Arch Dermatol 1945;51:370–372.

104. Goldstein N. Epidrosis (local hyperhidrosis), nevus sudoriferus. Arch Dermatol 1967;96:67–68.

105. Martius I: Lokalisierte ekkrine Schweissdrusenhyperlasie. Dermatol Monatsschr 1979;165:327–330.

106. Herzberg JJ: Ekkrine Syringocystadenom. Arch Klin Exp Dermatol 1962;214:600–621.

107. Hyman AB, Harris H, Brownstein MH. Eccrine angiomatous hamartoma. NY State J Med 1968;68:2803–2806.

108. Challa VR, Jona J. Eccrine angiomatous hamartoma: A rare skin lesion with diverse histological features. Dermatologica 1977;155:206–209.

109. Zeller DJ, Goldman RL. Eccrine-pilar angiomatous hamartoma. Dermatologica 1971;143:100–104.

110. Kikuchi I, Kuroki Y, Inoue S. Painful eccrine angiomatous nevus on the sole. J Dermatol 1982;9:329–332.

111. Mehregan AH: Proliferation of sweat ducts in certain diseases of the skin. Am J Dermatopathol 1981;3:27–31.

112. Santa Cruz DJ, Clausen K. Atypical sweat duct hyperplasia accompanying keratoacanthoma. Dermatologica 1977;154:156–160.

113. Farmer ER, Helwig EB. Cutaneous ciliated cysts. Arch Dermatol 1978;114:70–73.

114. Clark JV. Ciliated epithelium in a cyst of the lower limb. J Pathol 1969;98:289–290.

115. True L, Golitz LE. Ciliated plantar cyst. Arch Dermatol 1980;116:1066–1067.

116. Leonforte JE. Cutaneous ciliated cystadenoma in a man. Arch Dermatol 1980;118:1010–1012.

117. Hashimoto K, Gross BG, Lever WF. The ultrastructure of human embryo skin. II. The formation of intradermal portion of the eccrine sweat duct and of the secretory segment during the first half of embryonic life. J Invest Dermatol 1966;46:513–529.

118. Freeman RG, Winkelmann RK. Basal cell tumor with eccrine differentiation (eccrine epithelioma). Arch Dermatol 1969;100:234–242.

119. Sanchez NP, Winkelmann RK. Basal cell tumor with eccrine differentiation (eccrine epithelioma). J Am Acad Dermatol 1982;6:514–518.

120. Thomas JW, Fu YS, Levine MR. Primary mucinous sweat gland carcinoma of the eyelid simulating metastatic carcinoma. Am J Ophthalmol 1979;87:29–33.

121. Cohen KL, Peiffer RL, Lipper S. Mucinous sweat gland adenocarcinoma of the eyelid. Am J Ophthalmol 1981;92:183.

122. Wright JD, Font RL. Mucinous sweat gland adenocarcinoma of the eyelid. Cancer 1979;44:1757–1768.

123. Lahav M, Albert DM, Bahr R, Craft J. Eyelid tumors of sweat gland origin. Albrecht Arch Klin Exp Ophthalmol 1981;216:301–311.

124. Grossman JR, Izuno GT. Primary mucinous (adenocystic) carcinoma of the skin. Arch Dermatol 1974;110:274–276.

125. Yeung K-Y, Stinson JC. Mucinous (adenocystic) carcinoma of sweat glands with widespread metastasis. Cancer 1977;39:2556–2562.

126. Headington JT. Primary mucinous carcinoma of skin. Cancer 1977;39:1055–1063.

127. Santa Cruz DJ, Meyers JH, Gnepp DR, Perez BM. Primary mucinous carcinoma of the skin. Br J Dermatol 1978;98:645–653.
128. Mendoza S,. Helwig EB. Mucinous (adenocystic) carcinoma of the skin. Arch Dermatol 1971;103:68–78.
129. Lever WF, Schaumburg-Lever G. Histopathology of the skin. 6th edition, Philadelphia: JB Lippincott, 1983;6th ed, 560.
130. Kersting DW. Clear cell hidradenoma and hidradenocarcinoma. Arch Dermatol 1963;87:323–333.
131. Hernandez-Perez E, Cruz FA. Clear cell hidroadenocarcinoma: Report of an unusual case. Dermatologica 1976;153:249–252.
132. Headington JT, Niederhuber JE, Beals TF. Malignant clear cell acrospiroma. Cancer 1978;41:641–647.
133. El-Domeiri AA, Brasfield RD, Huvos AG, et al: Sweat gland carcinoma. Ann Surg 1971;173:270–274.
134. Boggio R. Adenoid cystic carcinoma of the scalp. Arch Dermatol 1975;111:793–794.
135. Headington JT, Tesars R, Niederhuber JE, et al. Primary adenoid cystic carcinoma of the skin. Arch Dermatol 1978;114:421–424.
136. Goslen JB, Eisen AZ, Bauer EA. Stimulation of skin fibroblast collagenase production by a cytokine derived from basal cell carcinomas. J Invest Dermatol 1985;85:161–164.
137. Goldstein DJ, Barr RJ, Santa Cruz DJ. Microcystic adnexal carcinoma: A distinct clinicopathologic entity. Cancer 1982;50:566–572.
138. Cooper PH. Sclerosing carcinomas of sweat ducts (microcystic adnexal carcinoma). Arch Dermatol 1986;122:261–264.
139. Nickoloff BJ, Fleischmann HE, Carnel J, et al. Microcystic adnexal carcinoma. Immunohistologic observations suggesting dual (pilar and eccrine) differentiation. Arch Dermatol 1986;122:290–294.
140. Lupton GP, McMarlin SL. Microcystic adnexal carcinoma. Report of a case with 30-year follow-up. Arch Dermatol 1986;122:286–289.

3

Hair Follicle Tumors

In early embryonic development hair germs emerge from the epidermis. The tip of the hair germ differentiates into the hair bulb and begins to produce a hair shaft and three layers of inner root sheath. The bulb's outer cells form the outer root sheath, which is continuous with the epidermis. Above the entry of the sebaceous duct into the hair follicle, the outer root sheath comes into direct contact with hair because the inner root sheath, which had protected incompletely keratinized hair below this level, undergoes complete keratinization and desquamates. The segment of the outer root sheath located between the entry of the sebaceous duct and the opening of the hair canal to the surface is called the *infundibulum*.

The infundibulum is keratinized in the same way as the epidermis: through the formation of stellate keratohyalin granules (Table 3.1). However, this segment of the hair follicle is a separate biologic entity; in actinic keratosis and large cell acanthoma, in which the surrounding epidermis is altered, the infundibulum is usually spared and appears sharply distinguished from the interfollicular epidermis.[1] The mitotic population of this unit may be spared the cumulative damages of actinic irradiation because it is located deeper than the interfollicular epidermis. The infundibulum has strong regenerative power, exemplified by the process of wound healing in which lost epidermis is often

Table 3.1
Mode of keratinization in different organs

Tissues	Formation of keratohyalin	None or minimal formation of keratohyalin
Epidermis	+ + +	
Outer root sheath		
Infundibulum	+ +	
Isthmus		±
Mucous membrane		
Gingiva, hard palate, tongue, cheek	+ +	
Soft palate, floor of the mouth		±
Hair shaft (cortex)		±
Inner root sheath	+ + +	
Nail		
Adult		−
Fetus	+ +	

replaced by a spread of infundibular keratinocytes. In vitiligo and scleroderma, repigmentation or retention of melanocytes is often seen in the follicular openings. Hyperplasia or faulty regeneration of the infundibulum produces several tumors, and various follicular neoplasms are assumed to arise from the follicular infundibulum.

Uniform diagnostic criteria applicable to all hair follicle tumors do not exist because the tumors vary so greatly depending on their degree of maturity and the follicular structures to which they are differentiating. However, glycogen-containing clear cells, a tendency to keratinize such as by forming keratin cysts (e.g., trichoepithelioma), trichilemmal keratinization, development of squamous eddies, hair germ-like or hair bulb-like budding of small basophilic cells, or hair formation are helpful hints. Ultrastructurally, the inner root sheath, cortex and outer hair sheath show their characteristic modes of keratinization (Table 3.1).

Tumor of the Follicular Infundibulum

This rare tumor occurs on the head and neck region of older individuals (aged 40 to 70).[2] Clinically, it is a single, 5- to 10-mm, smooth or slightly keratotic nodule that resembles a flat, seborrheic keratosis.

Histology

A plate of tumor is attached to the undersurface of the hyperkeratotic epidermis (Fig. 3.1). The plate is fenestrated by papillary connective tissue and capillaries. The interface between the stroma often shows palisading tumor cells and a thickened basement membrane. The tumor cells stain lightly and contain glycogen. Structures resembling hair follicles or hair germ-like buddings may be associated with it (Fig. 3.1A, B). When the hair follicle enters the tumor, the outer root sheath cells of the follicle cannot be clearly distinguished. This tumor may represent incompletely formed follicular epithelioma.[2,3]

Dilated Pore of Winer

This is a relatively common tumor often located in the head and neck region of individuals in all age groups.[2] It is usually a solitary lesion but occasionally occurs as multiple (2 to 3) nodules 4 to 10 mm in diameter.[2] It contains a central pore plugged with keratinous material.[4]

Histology
The funnel-shaped or balloon-like dilated follicular structure may be connected to a hair follicle at the lower end. The cystic space may be multilobulated (Fig. 3.2) and, in rare instances, the opening is widened in a dish-like fashion.[5] The tumor may stop at the level of the sebaceous gland or extend to the junction of the dermis and fat tissue.[6] The wall of the dilated pore exhibits finger-like projections, interdigitated deeply with dermal papillae, into the dermis. The pore's surface is completely keratinized through keratohyalin formation as occurs in infundibular keratinization. The keratin layer is usually thick. Desquamated keratin fills the pore (Fig. 3.2) and is clinically recognized as a keratin plug.

Pilar Sheath Acanthoma

This rare tumor always occurs on the face, most commonly on the upper lip of 40- to 70-year-old individuals.[2,7] A single skin-colored nodule (5 to 10 mm) contains a central pore, which may be either empty or plugged with keratin.

Histology
This is a more complicated neoplasm of the follicular infundibulum than the dilated pore of Winer; the cyst is connected to the surface[8] like a dilated pore, and the wall cells are light staining. Basal cells are palisaded, as in a tumor of the follicular infundibulum; however, in contrast to the dilated pore of Winer, the wall is much more acanthotic and more extensive epithelial projections extend from the wall into the surrounding stroma[9] (Fig. 3.3). Within this thick wall, pseudo or true horn cysts may be present. Some of the keratin cysts may represent secondary hair follicles, and thus, such feature places this tumor close to trichofolliculoma.[8]

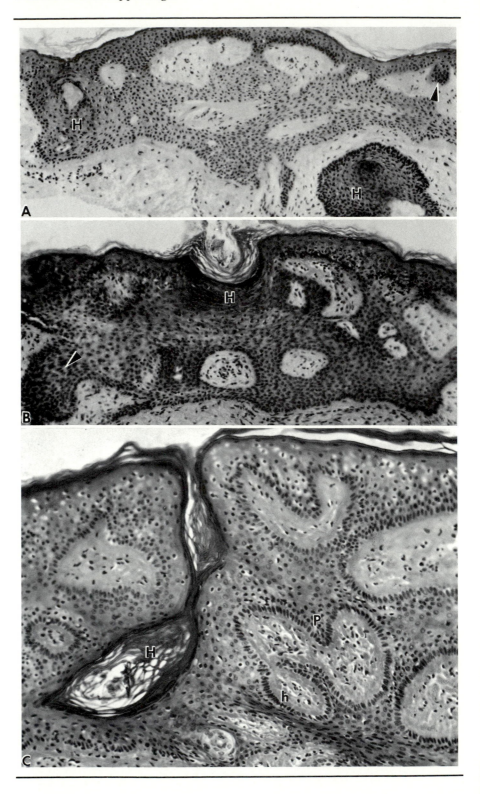

Figure 3.1
Tumor of follicular infundibulum. A horizontal epithelial plate is attached to the epidermis by several connecting points and between them are fenestrations of papillary dermis (A and B). The peripheral cells are small and basophilic and their nuclei are palisading (P) (C). Hair-like structures (H) and hair germ-like buddings (arrowheads) are seen (B). The basement membrane that envelops the epithelial strands is often hyalinized (h). The centrally located cells are large, pale, or clear and contain glycogen. (A and B, × 130; C, × 170.) (C is courtesy of Martin C. Mihm, Jr., M.D.)

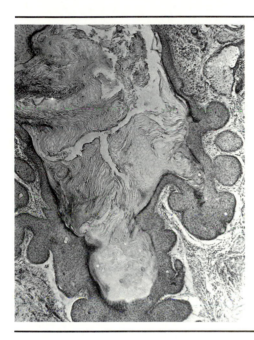

Figure 3.2
Dilated pore of Winer. A deep funnel-shaped dilated follicle contains a keratin plug. The follicular wall shows finger-like projections. (× 65.)

Trichofolliculoma

This tumor is a benign proliferation of hair roots and hair follicles and usually occurs on the face but also may arise on the scalp or neck. It is a dome-shaped lesion that may resemble basal cell epithelioma or keratoacanthoma because of its central depression or pore, out of which tufts of white woolly hairs may emerge.[10]

Histology
Clinically observed central depression or pore of the lesion is histologically a dilated follicular opening containing keratin plug and hairs. The lower portion of this "primary" follicle branches into multiple hair roots or "secondary" follicles (Fig. 3.4). Although every hair bulb-like structure seems to attempt to produce a hair, their differentiation usually stops at the hair cone stage

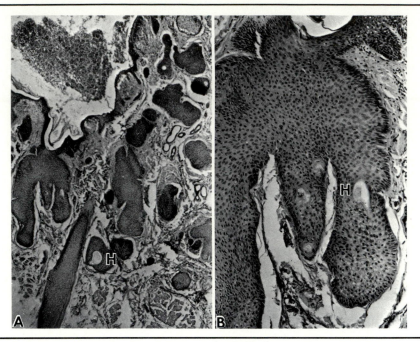

Figure 3.3
*Pilar sheath acanthoma. Its cystic dilated follicle, keratin plug, and finger-like pro-
jections* (A) *are similar to those of dilated pore of Winer (see Fig. 3.2). However,
these projections are more extensive and some resemble hair follicles* (B) *with abortive hair and hair canal formations* (H). (A, × 52; B, × 130.)

(Fig. 3.4D) and only a few bulbs form mature hairs. In some lesions the
proliferation of hair bulb structures is rather primitive, resembling basal cell
epithelioma or trichoepithelioma (Fig. 3.4E). Except for hair bulbs, most of
the tumor cells differentiate toward the outer root sheath and may appear
clear due to glycogen, which is present in varying amounts. The fibrous stroma
surrounding secondary follicles is well organized and is distinct from the adjacent dermal collagen bundles.

In *sebaceous trichofolliculoma,*[11] which occurs on the nose, numerous well-
differentiated sebaceous lobules and ducts are found as are a few hair structures (Fig. 3.4F). The clinical appearance of this variant is similar to that of
trichofolliculoma.

Fibrofolliculoma

The tumor consists of 2- to 4-mm firm papules with or without central hairs.
It usually occurs multiply and may be associated with trichodiscoma and
acrochordon[12,13] or with a large connective tissue nevus.[14]

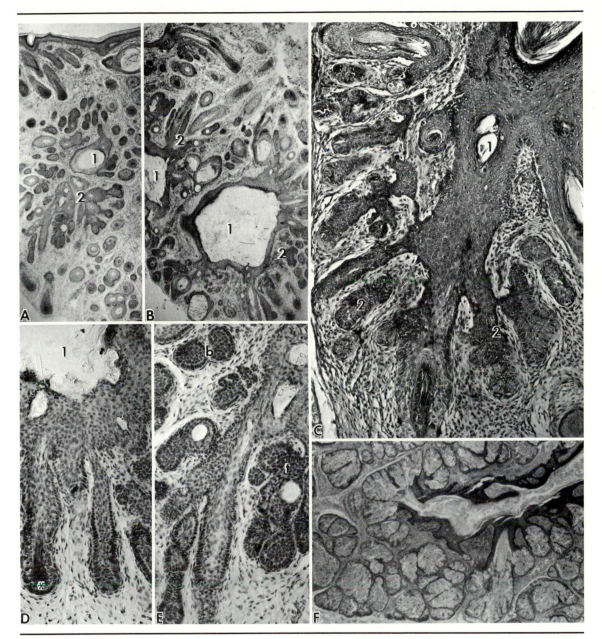

Figure 3.4
Trichofolliculoma. In A, B, and C, a large cystic space (primary follicle) (1) is surrounded by secondary follicles (2). In D and E, some secondary follicles are no more differentiated than those occasionally seen in basal cell epithelioma (b) or trichoepithelioma (t), but a few are fully mature and contain a hair cone (*). In F, sebaceous trichofolliculoma is shown. In this variety, the primary follicle is attached to numerous sebaceous glands. (A, B, and F, × 52; C, × 130; D and E, × 130.)

Histology

In the center is a dilated hair follicle from which thin, anastomosing strands of follicular epithelium extend outward into a well-organized fibrous or myxomatous stroma.

Trichilemmoma

This is a relatively common tumor of adults (ages 20 to 80).[2] The nose, upper lip, and other parts of the head and neck are exclusively affected. Usually a single 3- to 8-mm keratotic growth or a shiny, smooth papule is found. The exception is Cowden's disease, in which numerous papules cover the face, particularly the nose and upper lip.[15]

Histology

The well-defined growth extends from the epidermis (Fig. 3.5) and may be connected to an underlying pilosebaceous unit.[16] Tumor cells stain lightly and contain glycogen. The peripheral (basal) cells are palisading. The tumor epithelium is surrounded with a layer of diastase-resistant, PAS-positive hyalin material resembling the vitreous membrane of the hair follicles. Some tumors have a hair follicle-like configuration (Fig. 3.5B, C, E).

Cowden's Disease

Among the cutaneous manifestations of this autosomal dominant disease, multiple facial trichilemmomas have been considered its hallmark (Fig. 3.6). Breast cancer is the most important internal malignancy, reported in 29% of female patients[17]; other neoplasms are found in the thyroid and colon. Associated cutaneous lesions may include lichenoid and verrucous tumors of the hands and feet (acral keratoses) and punctate palmoplantar keratoses.[18] Oral lesions include smooth or keratotic papules, papillomatosis of the lips and oral mucosa, and scrotal tongue.[18]

Histology

Most facial biopsies reveal slight to marked hyperplasia of the follicular infundibulum (Fig. 3.5D, E), ranging from a tumor of the follicular infundibulum[3] to trichilemmoma.[18] Trichilemmoma may be cylindrical, resembling a blown-up hair follicle (Fig. 3.5B, C), or may occur as a wide, lobulated type (Fig. 3.5A) often extending from the hair follicle like a nodular basal cell epithelioma.[18] Verrucous lesions resemble acrochordon, digitated, or filiform verruca. Oral lesions are ordinary papillomas,[15,18] and facial and extrafacial lesions could be fibromas, which show interwoven fascicles of coarse and widely spaced collagen fibers.[19] In some fibromas the collagen is hyalinized.[19] Extrafacial lesions, which may be the presenting symptoms of the disease, resemble verruca vulgaris and acrokeratosis verruciformis. Histologically, these suggest

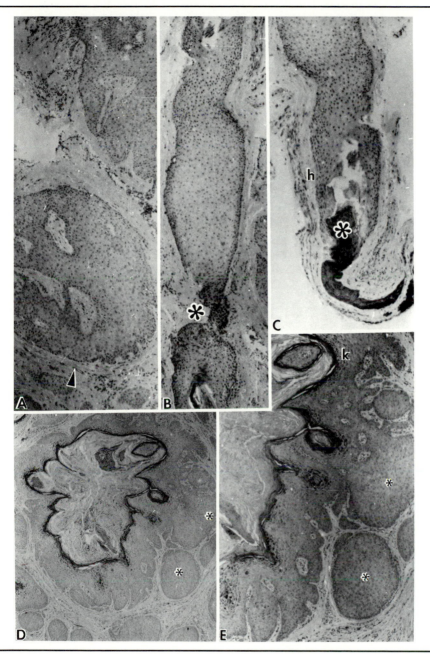

Figure 3.5
Trichilemmoma from a patient with Cowden's disease. In A, a lightly stained epithelial tumor extends from the epidermis down to a lobulated intradermal mass (arrowhead). In B and C tumors take the shape of a hair follicle (cylindrical type) and hair matrix (*). The peripheral (basal) cells are palisading, and perifollicular collagen is hyalinized (h). In D and E, the wall of a large follicular (infundibular) cyst is dedifferentiating into trichilemmoma (*). k—keratohyalin granules. (A, B, C, and E, ×
100; D, × 65.)

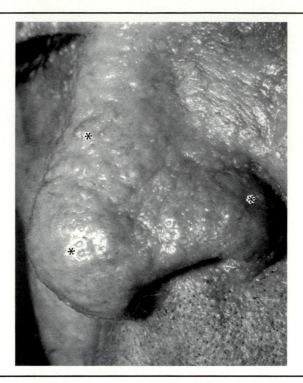

Figure 3.6
Cowden's disease. Facial lesions are small papules (*) that tend to aggregate and which may be mistaken for flat warts.

cylindrical trichilemmoma or inverted follicular keratosis[17]; however, many of the extrafacial lesions have the clinical as well as histologic appearance of warts. Bovine papillomavirus type I antigen is negative in both facial trichilemmoma and extrafacial wart-like lesions.[17,18]

Inverted Follicular Keratosis

This is a relatively common appendage tumor of adults (ages 30 to 70), which occurs in the head and neck region in 90% of the cases,[2,20,21] although some lesions may be found on the trunk and extremities. Clinically it is a single filiform, verrucous or hyperkeratotic nodular lesion. Occasionally the lesion has a smooth surface or is centrally umbilicated.[2]

Histology
Four major patterns are recognized: papillomatous or wart-like, keratoacanthoma-like, solid nodular type, and cystic type.[2] In all forms, layers of small basaloid cells line the periphery of the tumor masses. In the thick epithelial mass or the follicle-like structure, the central portion becomes more squamoid

and eosinophilic with concentric layers of cells forming "squamous eddies" (Fig. 3.7C, E, F). Basaloid cells are usually admixed with squamoid cells and squamous eddies, or tend to aggregate together (Figs. 3.7B, C). Although connection with an underlying pilosebaceous unit can occasionally be demonstrated (Fig. 3.7D), it is sometimes difficult to separate this lesion from an irritated seborrheic keratosis. A group of small basaloid cells that may be found surrounding the squamous eddies certainly resembles those observed in seborrheic keratosis. In some lesions a large number of dendritic melanocytes are admixed as in melanoacanthoma, a variant of seborrheic keratosis. Thus, opinions are divided whether inverted follicular keratosis should be considered a distinct tumor[21] or an irritated seborrheic keratosis involving the follicular epithelium.[22]

Eruptive Vellus Hair Cyst

The tumor usually appears on the chest as multiple papules.[23] The surface may be smooth, crusted, or umbilicated. Young adults are commonly affected and spontaneous resolution may occur. Autosomal dominant inheritance has been reported.[24,25] In the rare facial variant described by Kumakiri et al.[26] in Japanese patients over age 50, asymptomatic, slate-colored maculopapules are disseminated mainly over the forehead. In colored skin even the chest lesions appear bluish to slate colored; therefore, slate color of the facial variant is probably not specific.

Trichostasis spinulosa may simulate eruptive vellus hair cyst histologically because a number of vellus hairs are present in dilated follicles. Clinically, however, trichostasis spinulosa affects the back; the interscapular area in particular is often pruritic and shows bundled vellus hairs growing out of hyperkeratotic follicles.

Histology

A cystic hair follicle containing many vellus hairs is found in the mid-dermis (Fig. 3.8). In crusted or umbilicated lesions, the cyst wall either communicates with the surface or is being destroyed by a foreign body-type granulomatous reaction within the surrounding connective tissue. The wall of the cyst may be infundibular or trichilemmal; in the latter, typical trichilemmal keratinization (Table 3.1) is seen on electron microscopy.[26] Small hairs may emerge from the the wall[26,27] (Fig. 3.8F, G).

Nevus Comedonicus

This is a congenital malformation or nevoid lesion of the pilosebaceous unit that develops in childhood, adolescence, or later in life. It usually shows a linear, unilateral arrangement of dark, keratotic plugs; hence the name nevus unilateralis comedonicus. Several other variants include multiple or linear bilateral lesions,[28] localized nonlinear lesions,[29] and plantar and palmar involve-

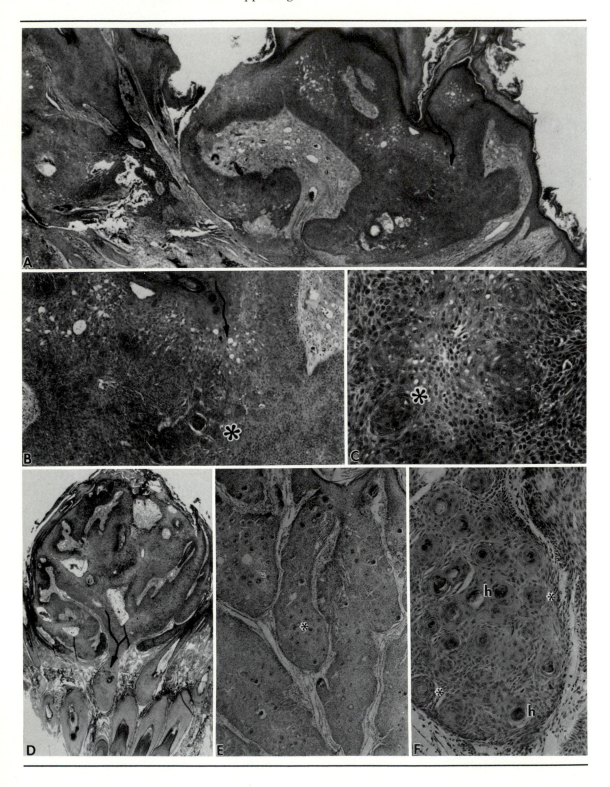

Figure 3.7
Inverted follicular keratosis. A verrucous exophytic growth forms a pear-shaped epithelial mass that can be traced to an underlying hair follicle (arrows) (A, B, and D). The composition of this tumor with small basophilic cells is similar to seborrheic keratosis except for the concentric aggregations of squamoid cells (squamous eddies) (*) (B, C, and E) that resemble horn pearls (h) in shape and size (F). Squamous eddies (*) are diagnostic. B and C were taken from the tumor shown in A, and E and F from D. (A and D, × 31; B and E, × 61; C, × 156; F, × 56.)

ment, either in addition to lesions on other parts[30] or limited to palm[31] or sole.[32] The palmar and plantar lesions are related to eccrine sweat duct nevus (see porokeratotic eccrine ostial and dermal duct nevus, p. 25), representing overlapping of a nevoid condition of the hair follicle and eccrine gland.

Histology
Individual lesions represent keratin-plugged hair follicles (Fig. 3.9); at the bottom of the dilated follicle there may be one or several hairs.[29] In early lesions, small sebaceous glands are present connected to the wall.[29] The wall cells undergo an outer root sheath type of keratinization (Table 3.1). Several instances of vacuolar degeneration of granular cells[33] or sebaceous ducts,[34] similar to that seen in epidermolytic hyperkeratosis, have been reported. In this regard the condition may be related to ichthyosis hystrix.

Trichoadenoma

This tumor arises in the outer root sheath of the hair follicle.[35,36] A solitary dermal nodule of 3 to 15 mm usually occurs on the face but may also appear on the trunk. There is no age preference.

Histology
Multiple cystic spaces are lined with outer root sheath epithelium containing keratohyalin granules. This mode of keratinization is also compatible with that of the follicular infundibulum (Table 3.1), and in fact the tumor appears to be composed of multiple empty hair canals (Fig. 3.10). Although there is no hair root formation, in some tumors or in parts of typical lesions a short epithelial cord is attached to the wall of the cyst (Fig. 3.10B, D). If this phenomenon is prevalent, the lesion may simulate a trichoepithelioma (see Fig. 3.18A, B). A fibrous stroma surrounds the cystic structures.

Steatocystoma Multiplex

This is an autosomal dominant disease that affects both sexes. Onset is usually postadolescence when pilosebaceous units are active. The patient complains

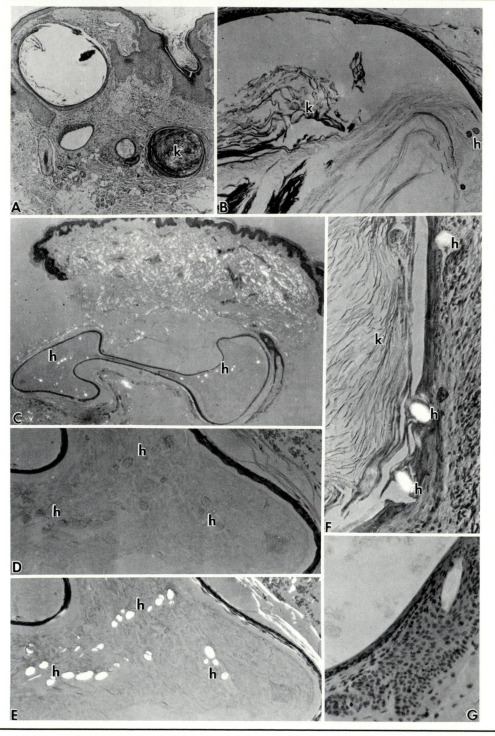

Figure 3.8

Eruptive vellus hair cyst. Intradermal cysts contain keratin (k) and hair (h). Under polarized light the hairs become birefringent (C, E, and F); D is viewed under polarized light to yield birefringent hairs in E. It is seen in F that hairs are incorporated into the cyst wall. In G, even hair follicle-like differentiation of the wall is seen. (A and C, × 52; B, D, and E, × 130; F and G, × 163.)

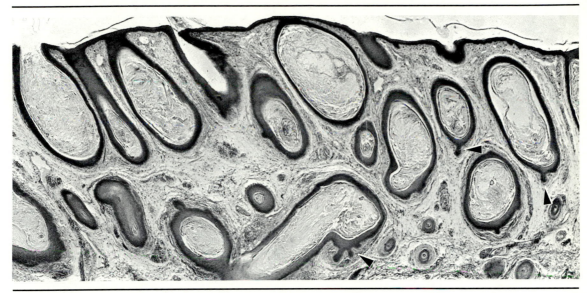

Figure 3.9
Nevus comedonicus. Most of the keratin cysts are open to the surface; a few are enclosed within the dermis. There are several buds (arrowheads) from the wall of the cysts, but there is no hair follicle formation in this specimen. (× 65.)

of a gradually increasing number of small intradermal nodules (1 to 3 cm) mainly on the sternum, the axillae, the upper arms, and the scrotum. Multiple scrotal cysts may or may not be associated with the condition. In rare instances large (up to 3 cm), multiple, deeply seated tumors cover almost the entire body, often in chains.[37,38] Most of these giant tumors are steatocystoma, although epidermoid cysts may also be present. The solitary, nonhereditary variety is known as steatocystoma simplex.[39] The content of steatocystoma is liquid or oily and odorless, in contrast to epidermoid or trichilemmal cyst, which contains semi-solid, rancid material, often referred to as cheesy materials.

Histology
Infolded narrow cystic spaces lie parallel to each other. It is likely that many projections or growths from the cyst wall into the central cavity are compressed into slender septae and divide the cavity into intricately connected thin slits (Fig. 3.11C, D). The wall consists of several layers of cells in thick portions and only two or three cell layers in atrophic areas. In average areas, palisading basal cells transform into large squamoid cells that eventually flatten and line the cyst cavity. The mode of keratinization is trichilemmal[39,40] (Table 3.1). The luminal cells have a corrugated surface and often retain their nucleus (Fig. 3.11A). When the plane of section is tangential to the lumen, these corrugated cells are cut like interrupted ribbons (Fig. 3.11A), suggesting that the surface is undulating. Epidermoid keratinization may occur in thick areas of the wall.

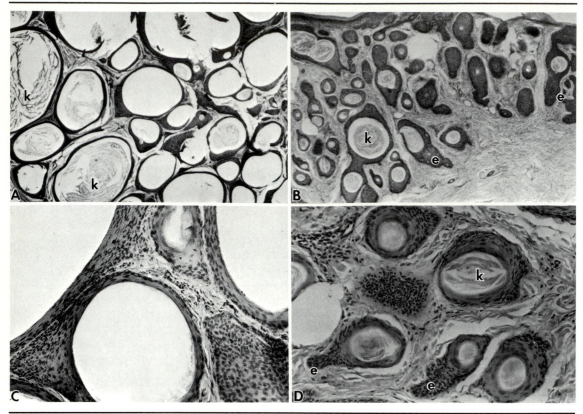

Figure 3.10
Trichoadenoma. Multiple epithelial cysts, lined with follicular sheath epithelium containing keratin shells (k), are evident (A and C). Some cysts are attached to a short epithelial cord (e) (B and D) and appear similar to trichoepithelioma. There is no hair matrix or actual hair formation. (A and B, × 65; C and D, × 130.)

In contrast to trichilemmal or epidermoid cysts, the lumen is devoid of content (Fig. 3.11). During tissue processing it is likely that the lipid contents[41] are dissolved in alcohol and xylene. The most helpful diagnostic feature of this tumor is the presence of sebaceous glands that are either incorporated into the wall or attached to it (Fig. 3.11B, C, D). Thin hair shafts may be found in the cyst, where small hair follicles project into the surrounding stroma. The direction of differentiation with this tumor seems to be toward the sebaceous gland—isthmus portion of the hair follicle. The normal sebaceous duct undergoes keratinization with formation of keratohyalin. Although such areas may be seen in thick portions of the cyst wall, most of the epithelial wall does not show this feature.

Trichilemmal Cyst

This term has replaced the old one, "sebaceous cyst," since Pinkus redefined the lesion.[42] There is no true "sebaceous cyst," that is, a cyst composed of

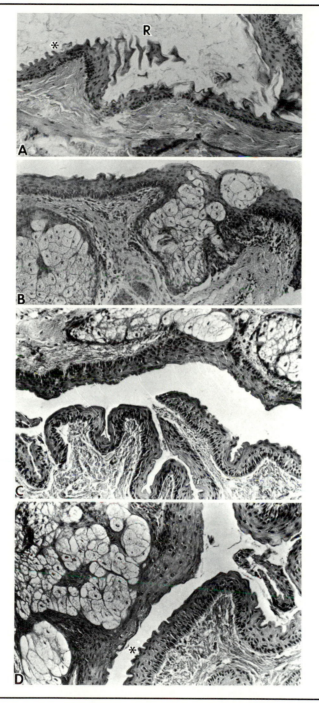

Figure 3.11
Steatocystoma multiplex. The wall of the cyst is composed of small basal cells, large squamoid cells, and incompletely keratinized surface cells that show undulated or corrugated surfaces (* in A and D). When such an undulated surface is sectioned tangentially, a ribbon of interrupted keratin is produced (R in A). The sebaceous glands incorporated in the wall (B, C, and D) help to differentiate steatocystoma from a trichilemmal cyst. The cystic space may be divided into many invaginations by an infolding cyst wall (C and D). (A and B, × 100; C and D, × 165.)

sebaceous glands: only a part of the cyst in steatocystoma multiplex is composed of sebaceous gland (Fig. 3.11). The term is probably attributable to the sebum-like or cheesy contents of these cysts.

The majority (90%) of trichilemmal cysts are found on the scalp; a few appear in other locations. Multiple trichilemmal cysts may occur. An autosomal mode of inheritance is established.[43]

Histology

Basal cells in the lining of the cyst wall are distinctive because they are palisading and are densely basophilic. They are much smaller than the large, swollen eosinophilic cells above them (Fig. 3.12A, B, C). The larger squamoid cells accumulate glycogen and become clear and balloon-like but retain their

Figure 3.12
Trichilemmal cyst. In A, B, and C only two types of cells are seen: palisading basal cells (arrowheads) and large ballooning cells that shed into the cyst without forming keratohyalin granules. In E, a polarized light view of D is shown: near the wall keratin birefringence is more intense than toward the center of the cyst. (A and B, × 163; C, × 520; D and E, × 100.)

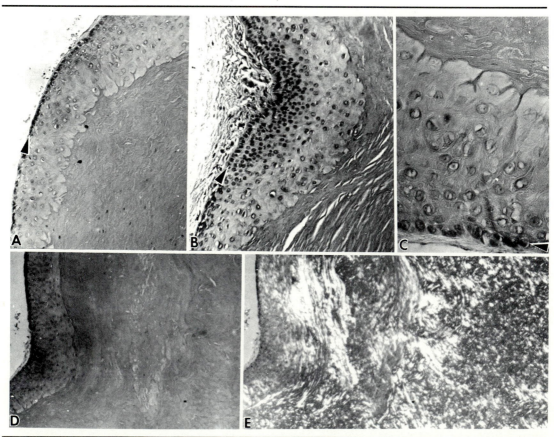

nuclei (Fig. 3.12C). These large balloon cells undergo keratinization, lose their nuclei, and shed into a homogeneous eosinophilic material within the cystic cavity. Occasionally, small areas of keratohyalin granules may be produced. Under polarized light the cyst content near the wall is strongly birefringent because keratin fibers are still intact, whereas birefringence is diminished or absent toward the center of the cyst (Fig. 3.12D, E). Calcification is frequently seen in trichilemmal cysts but rarely in epidermoid cysts.

Electron Microscopy

Large balloon cells protruding into the cyst contain, in addition to glycogen, numerous vesicles, vacuoles, and dense vesicular bodies (Fig. 3.13A, C). Multivesicular dense bodies, some of which are laminated, are membrane bound and discharge into the intercellular spaces (Fig. 3.13C). These findings suggest that they are a multivesicular type of lysosome and as such represent modified lamellar bodies (*i.e.,* Odland body, membrane-coating granule, cementsome, etc.). Recent work indicates that the epidermal lamellar bodies contain most of the lysosomal enzymes in addition to phospholipids, free sterols, and glycosphingolipids.[44,45] Small keratohyalin granules are present even in those balloon cells that do not appear to contain keratohyalin on light microscopy (Fig. 3.13C). Sparse bundles of tonofilaments and dense ground matrix fill the rest of the cytoplasm (Fig. 3.13A). These organelles are very similar to those found in the follicular isthmus[46,47] (Fig. 3.13B) and in the lower sac surrounding club hairs of catagen and telogen follicles.[48] The cyst is therefore considered to represent a proliferation of epithelium from the follicular isthmus or telogen hair sac. This epithelium produces incompletely keratinized material in quantity, and if by some accident the follicular orifice is occluded (this may be the primary cause), an expanding tumor or cyst may form.

In other instances, follicular occlusion may produce an *epidermoid cyst* in which the follicular infundibulum is one of the possible sources of proliferation (another is posttraumatic inclusion of the epidermis) (Fig. 3.14). In epidermoid cysts the wall is composed of stratified layers of basal, squamoid (prickle), granular, and horny cells as in the surface epidermis or follicular infundibulum (Fig. 3.14). In some cysts DOPA-positive melanocytes are present in the basal layer (Fig. 3.14E). In rare instances the lower part of the cyst wall is trichilemmal and the upper part is an epidermoid, that is, a hybrid cyst[49] (Fig. 1.3); a follicular origin of such cysts is beyond any doubt. *Facial milium* is a simple occlusion of the upper hair follicle, and the wall consists of outer root sheath epithelium (Fig. 3.15).

Proliferating Trichilemmal Cyst (Tumor) or Pilar Tumor

This tumor, reported under several different names,[50–52] represents a proliferative variant of the trichilemmal cyst. It usually occurs in elderly women as a solitary tumor on the scalp[53] and occasionally elsewhere.[54] It begins as a subcutaneous nodule but gradually becomes exophytic and eventually may

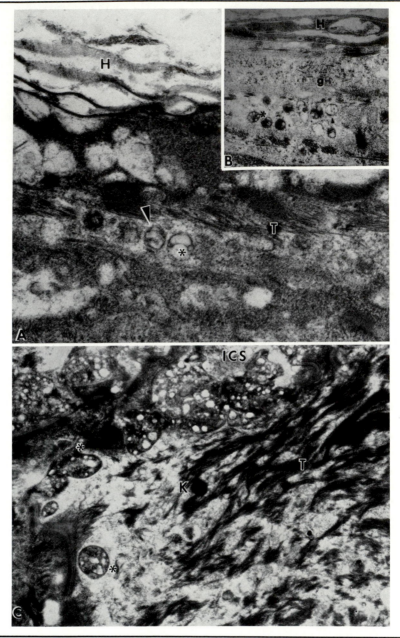

Figure 3.13
Trichilemmal cyst. In A, electron microscopy reveals large ballooning cells near the cyst border that contain multivesicles (*), laminated bodies (arrowhead), tonofilaments (T), and dense cytoplasm. These cells become flat horny cells (H) without forming keratohyalin granules. B is a very similar picture of the normal follicular infundibulum; g indicates glycogen. H indicates incompletely keratinized horny cells. In C another area of the cyst wall contains predominantly multivesicular bodies and no laminated bodies. These vesicular bodies are delimited with membrane. They fuse with the cell membrane and discharge the contents into intercellular spaces (ICS). One keratohyalin granule (K) and sparse bundles of tonofilaments (T) are seen. (A and C, × 10,000; B, × 6,000.)

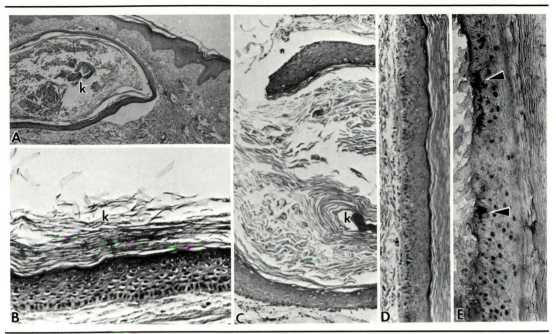

Figure 3.14
Epidermoid cyst. In contrast to a trichilemmal cyst (Fig. 3.12), the cyst wall is identical to the epidermis, and the cyst's laminated shells of keratin (k) are composed of mature epidermal keratin (A and C). Rete ridges are not formed (B and D). In some cysts the basal layer of the cyst wall contains DOPA-positive melanocyte (arrowheads in E). (A, × 52; B, × 150; C, × 100; D and E, × 130.)

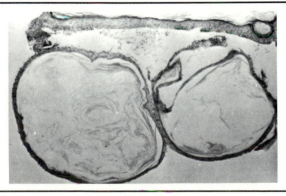

Figure 3.15
Facial milia. Two cystic spaces are lined by epidermoid wall cells and contain completely keratinized shells of keratin. (× 33.)

ulcerate. It may coexist with a regular trichilemmal cyst. Malignant transformation with lymph node metastasis has been reported, but the prognosis seems to be favorable.[55]

Histology

In some specimens or in some parts of the tumor there is a massive proliferation of outer root sheath epithelium with large eosinophilic cells, often exhibiting nuclear atypia and resembling an invasive squamous cell carcinoma (Fig. 3.16). However, multiple cysts filled with incompletely formed keratin and a trichilemmal mode of keratinization in other parts indicate that the tumor is related to the trichilemmal cyst. Glycogen-laden, large, clear cells in the tumor and occasional calcification of cyst contents further support this interpretation. A hyalin membrane may surround the periphery of the tumor parenchyma as it is along the lower portion of telogen (club) hair.

Trichoepithelioma

A multiple, autosomal dominant type and solitary, nonhereditary form have been recognized. In the multiple variety, dome-shaped, semitransparent small nodules (0.2 to 0.8 cm) appear on the face in childhood and may spread to the scalp, neck, and upper trunk. In children it may be clinically mistaken for

Figure 3.16
Proliferating trichilemmal cyst. In A and B, massive trichilemmal proliferation (T) coexists with large squamoid cells (*) similar to those seen in squamous cell carcinoma grade I. Hyperchromatism and atypia can be detected in C. In more benign areas palisading peripheral cells as in trichilemmoma can still be seen (arrowheads in D). (A, × 65; B, × 613; C, × 130; D, × 140.)

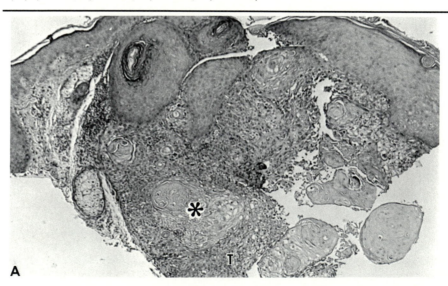

A

molluscum contagiosum. In some cases only sporadic lesions develop, but in most patients numerous lesions appear in the nasolabial folds, preauricular areas, and forehead. In severe cases these become confluent (Fig. 3.17A, B, C). Large, longstanding lesions may show superficial ulceration.[56] Coexistence with cylindroma has been recognized and considered an indication of apocrine or pilosebaceous differentiation of cylindroma.

The solitary type also occurs most commonly on the face but appears later in life. Solitary lesions are usually larger (up to 2 cm) than individual lesions of the multiple type (Fig. 3.17D). Apocrine adenoma may coexist in the same tumor.[57] The solitary variety is often misdiagnosed as basal cell epithelioma,

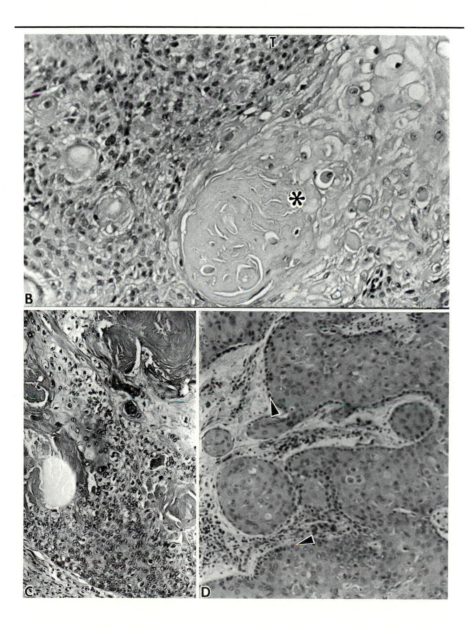

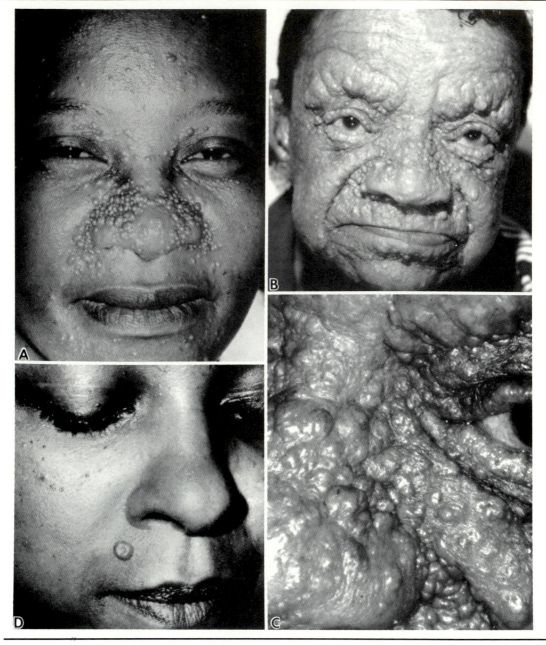

Figure 3.17
Trichoepithelioma. The moderately severe multiple type shows predilection for involvement on the nasolabial folds (A), *while the very severe multiple type covers literally the entire face* (B) *with a heavy concentration on the nasolabial fold* (C). *The solitary type* (D) *may resemble basal cell epithelioma; however, a young black individual is a very unlikely case for that.*

particularly when basaloid epithelial proliferation is dominant and cyst formation is minimal (Fig. 3.18D, E). Basal cell epithelioma in a young black patient is histologically a solitary trichoepithelioma in most instances (Fig. 3.17D).

Histology

Both multiple and solitary types show the same histologic features. The degree of maturation toward the pilar structures varies from very primitive (hair bulb-like) or basal cell epithelioma-like structures (Fig. 3.18D, E) to development of abortive hair follicles and horn cysts (Fig. 3.18A, B, C); these lesions may closely resemble trichoadenoma (Fig. 3.9, 3.10). Predominantly horn cyst lesions justify the old name *epithelioma adenoides cysticum,* whereas those in which hair bulbs and primitive epithelial buds dominate may be identical to the *trichoblastoma-trichogenic trichoblastoma* group (see Fig. 3.20).

Lesions in which basaloid cells predominate (Fig. 3.18E) are often difficult to differentiate from true basal cell epithelioma without clinical information. Such tumors may resemble all varieties of basal cell epithelioma, that is, branching, lace-like, adenoid, or sclerotic (in desmoplastic trichoepithelioma). Absence of horn cysts in basal cell epithelioma may help with the differentiation, but the so-called keratotic basal cell epithelioma may show a horn cyst. Helpful findings include admixture of fibroblasts within the parenchyma, small pocket-like invaginations of stroma into the parenchyma, and frequently sclerotic fibrous sheaths (Fig. 3.18E), instead of liquefaction of collagen, surrounding the tumor islands of trichoepithelioma. The fibrous tumor stroma may retract and separate from the surrounding dermis (Fig. 3.18E).

Some of the solid epithelial islands may represent abortive hair shaft (cortex) formation if they show large eosinophilic cells and a small aggregation of small basophilic cells representing development of a hair matrix (Fig. 3.18B). Abortive hair formation is also seen (Fig. 3.18B, C). Calcification may be found in these hair-related structures as well as in the keratin content of large cysts (see Fig. 3.19A, B, D). Other cysts may show distinct keratohyalin formation and completely keratinized cells similar to those of infundibular or epidermal keratinization; this type of cyst often contains hair (Fig. 3.18C). The majority of the cysts are lined with an incompletely keratinized wall and contain poorly stained keratinous debris (Fig. 3.18B); these cysts represent an isthmus type of differentiation. Electron microscopy demonstrates sparse small keratohyalin granules and incompletely keratinized wall cells.

Desmoplastic Trichoepithelioma

This tumor almost always occurs on the face of young women.[58,59] It is a solitary, firm nodule less than 1.0 cm in diameter with a central depression, appearing similar to a small granuloma annulare lesion.[36]

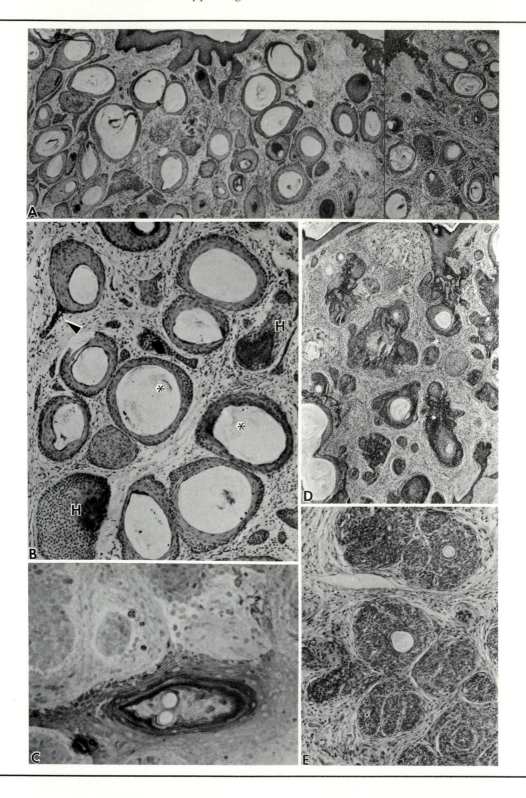

Figure 3.18
Trichoepithelioma. In A, multiple cysts are present on the left, and the mixture of cysts and epithelial components on the right are of the same specimen. In B, the cyst wall is incompletely keratinized and has shed into the cyst and is seen as poorly stained keratinous debris (*). A cyst has an epithelial cord (arrowhead); such cords may also be seen alone. Hair matrix-like differentiation is detected (H). In C a completely keratinized cyst wall and hairs are seen. In D and E, basaloid epithelial cell components predominate; except for the fibrotic stroma, these pictures closely resemble keratotic basal cell epithelioma. (A and D, × 33; B and E, × 130; C, × 200.)

Histology

Thin strands and small nests of basaloid cells are embedded in a markedly sclerotic stroma (Fig. 3.19). Some strands appear to be connected to acrosyringium and such feature raises the question whether some of the cysts may represent syringoma-like eccrine ductal differentiation (Fig. 3.19E). Occasionally, tadpole-like structures similar to those seen in syringoma are present (Fig. 3.19F, G). Other strands may be connected to the wall of keratin-filled horn cyst. Sebaceous glands may be embedded in the cyst wall suggesting that they originate from hair follicles (Fig. 3.19D). Calcification of keratin contents is seen in these cysts, sometimes associated with a foreign body granuloma (Fig. 3.19A, B, D). The stromal collagen is sclerotic and is organized parallel to the epithelial strands and surrounding the cyst walls. Organized stromal collagen is also present in sclerosing basal cell epithelioma and, therefore, if multiple cysts are not present, it may be difficult to differentiate this tumor from the morphea-like basal cell epithelioma (Fig. 3.19C).

Trichoblastoma and Trichoblastic Fibroma

These tumors, unlike solitary trichoepithelioma, occur anywhere except in the distal extremities.[60,61] The lesion is a solitary, firm subcutaneous or intradermal nodule. When one tries to remove the subcutaneous tumor it "shells out" easily, while intradermal tumors are firmly bound to the surrounding tissue. Male/female distribution is about equal. The size of the tumor varies from a few millimeters to several centimeters.[61] There is no familial background.

Histology

Although the histologic pattern shows considerable variation, it is common to see slender interlacing columns of basaloid epithelium, often only two cells thick (Fig. 3.20A, B). Differentiation of hair ranges from primitive germinal buds and solid columns to fully developed hair follicles containing hair shafts[59] (*trichogenic trichoblastoma*). Small keratinizing foci with or without cyst formation are present. Foci of sebaceous differentiation are observed in some tumors or in different areas of the same lesion (Fig. 3.20). The periphery of the tumor nodule or lobule is enveloped by fibrous stroma, which may form a major bulk of the tumor and which can be mucinous (Fig. 3.20C, E).

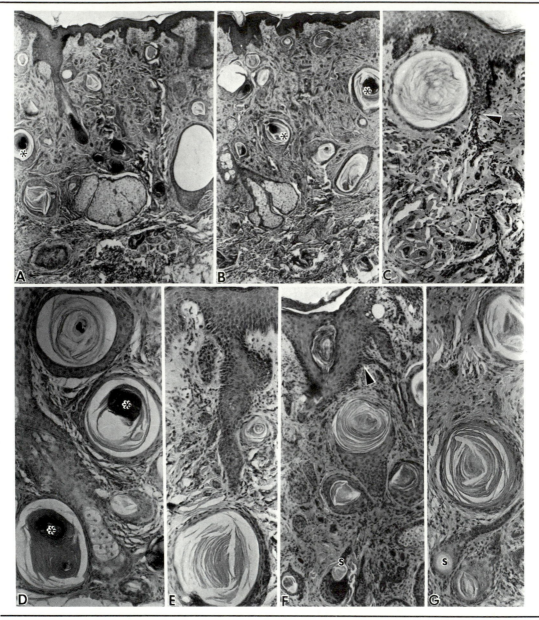

Figure 3.19
Desmoplastic trichoepithelioma. Multiple cysts containing calcified keratin (in A,
B, and D) are mixed with thin epithelial cords (A, B, and C). Some of these cords
are connected to the epidermis (arrowheads in C and F), while some other cysts,
such as seen in E, may be connected with eccrine duct. Tadpole-like structures (s)
commonly seen in syringoma are also present (F and G). Some cysts are apparently
attached with sebaceous gland (D). (A and B, × 33; C–G, × 65.)*

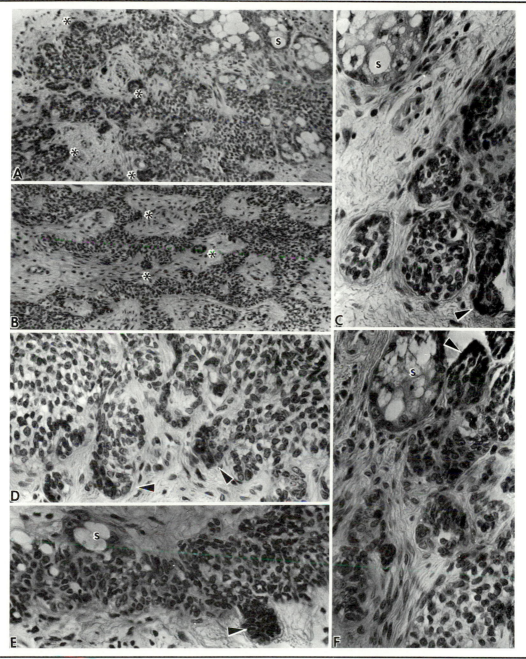

Figure 3.20
Trichoblastoma. In A and B, thin strands of basalioma-like epithelial growths anastomose to each other. Dense buds (*) and sebaceous differentiation (s in A, C, E, F) distinguish these from ordinary basal cell epithelioma. In C–F these buds appear similar to hair germs (arrowheads). The stroma is partially mucinous in C and E. (A and B, × 33; C–F, × 163.) (Courtesy of Thomas M. Chesney, M.D.)

Pilomatricoma (Calcifying Epithelioma of Malherbe)

This tumor represents a neoplasm of the hair matrix cell with relatively low grade cortical differentiation. Other cell components of the hair matrix, such as the inner root sheath and cuticles, may be present as minor components. As illustrated in Figures 1.2 and 3.22C, in rare instances a distinct follicular structure is present. Such a tumor may be clinically visible as a hyperkeratotic nodule. The majority of pilomatricomas are deep seated, stone hard, and lobulated (Fig. 3.21A, B). When the circumference of the growth is pressed with fingers, hard contents of the tumor may emerge like an iceberg or pitched tent (tent sign) (Fig. 3.21B). Pilomatricoma occurs predominantly on the face of young individuals, particularly children, as a single lesion. Multiple lesions are occasionally seen (Fig. 3.21A) and a hereditary type that is associated with myotonic dystrophy is also recognized.[62]

Histology

At low magnification, it is a well-circumscribed tumor in the deep dermis composed of eosinophilic areas, patchy aggregates of densely basophilic cells, and in most cases foci of foreign body granuloma in the stroma (Fig. 3.22A). In more organized tumors the periphery of the hair follicle-like structures is basophilic and toward the center acellular eosinophilic keratinous material accumulates and forms hair-like columns (Figs. 1.2 and 3.22C, E). However, in the majority of hair-like structures the center is filled with keratinous debris (Fig. 3.22D) instead of well-formed hair fibers. Calcification begins in the eosinophilic keratin. Foreign body reaction is elicited where the eosinophilic keratin is exposed to the connective tissue stroma. At high magnification basaloid cells may vary in size and in density of staining; those cells located at the periphery are small, basaloid, and densely basophilic, whereas those toward the center gradually become larger, acquire eosinophilic staining, and finally lose their nuclei. These terminally differentiated cells maintain their borders but their nuclei are recognized only as empty holes. These cells are called "shadow cells" (Fig. 3.22B).

Electron Microscopy

If one follows the transformation of basophilic cells to large squamoid cells to shadow cells and to amorphous keratin by electron microscopy, the basaloid cells are immature hair (cortex) cells that have not yet produced a significant amount of hair keratin fibers in their cytoplasm (Fig. 3.23A); they gradually become large squamoid cells whose cytoplasm is filled with aggregated keratin fibers[63] (Fig. 3.23B). Shadow cells represent the more mature keratinized hair cells in which the nucleus and other cellular organelles have disappeared under the pressure of accumulated keratin fibers or by programmed death after attaining terminal differentiation (Fig. 3.23C). The transition from large eosinophilic cells to shadow cells corresponds to the keratogenous zone of the anagen hair.

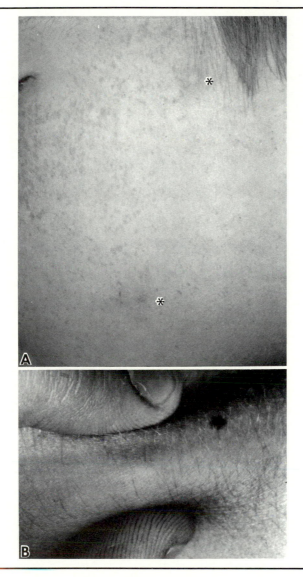

Figure 3.21
Pilomatricoma. In A, two lesions (*) on the cheek of this young boy are barely discernible because the lesions are so deep. In B, such a deep lesion was made visible by pinching it; the stone hard tumor emerged like an iceberg or pitched tent.

Basaloid Follicular Hamartoma

This condition can be generalized, linear, unilateral, or localized. Brown et al.[64] reported a 32-year-old black woman with myasthenia gravis who from the age of about 20 progressively lost her entire body hair. Ridley and Smith[65] reported a 32-year-old white woman with myasthenia gravis since age 16 who

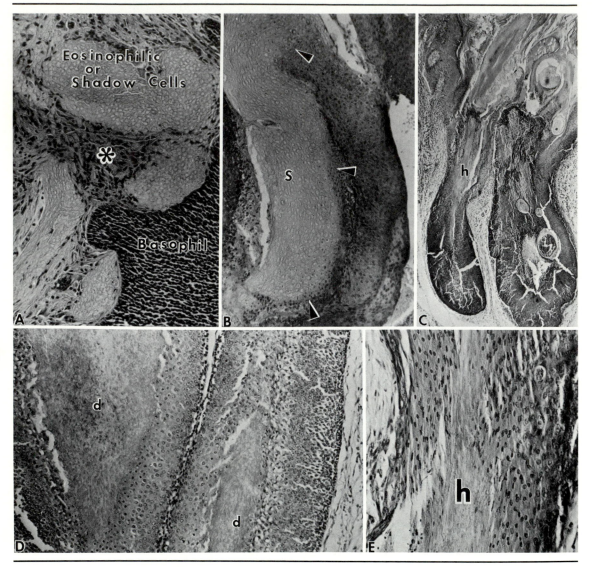

Figure 3.22

Pilomatricoma. In A, basophilic cells, eosinophilic or shadow cells, and a foreign body granuloma (*) coexist but are sharply divided. In B, basophilic cells are gradually transformed into shadow cells (S) by the loss of their nucleus (arrowheads). The column of shadow cells represents incompletely formed hair. In C, more completely formed hair (h) is seen toward the center and is magnified in E. Although these hair follicle-like structures are connected to the epidermis, they are entirely composed of hair (cortex) cells and are devoid of inner and outer root sheath; they represent the naked hair matrix. In D, the hair formation is abortive and shadow cells degenerate into amorphous debris (d). (A, B, and D, × 130; C, × 65; E, × 163.) (Courtesy of Akinobu Shoji, M.D., and Toshio Hamada, M.D.)

developed, for 18 months, an increasing area of erythematous infiltrated plaques and papular lesions on the face. Progressive hair loss eventually affected all other areas of the body including eyelashes and the anterior hair line of the scalp. Linear[66,67–69] or macular[70] varieties may occur in unilateral distribution with hypo- or hyperpigmentation.[70] Comedones or keratotic plugs are often seen in the lesions, thus, clinically, nevus unilateralis comedonicus or systematized epidermal nevus should be differentiated. The localized form may occur in the scalp, manifested as a plaque of alopecia.[70] The condition may be either congenital[66] or late in onset.[70]

Histology

In all varieties there are essentially three histologic components: (1) basal cell epithelioma-like or premalignant fibroepithelial tumor-like epithelial prolif-

Figure 3.23
Pilomatricoma. In A, basophilic cells as defined by the light microscopy are similar to the matrix cells of hair cortex. These are small, immature keratinocytes with wispy keratin fibrils (k) and prominent nucleoli (n). They are connected to each other with poorly developed desmosomes (arrowheads). In B, more developed, larger basophilic cells still retain their nucleus (N) and contain more prominent bundles of keratin fibrils (K). In C, the shadow cell's nucleus (N) has degenerated leaving only the nuclear membrane (arrowhead). Keratin fibrils are coalesced (K) and occupy a large area of these cells. Calcification (Ca) is noticed. (A, × 5,400; B, × 10,000; C, × 20,000.)

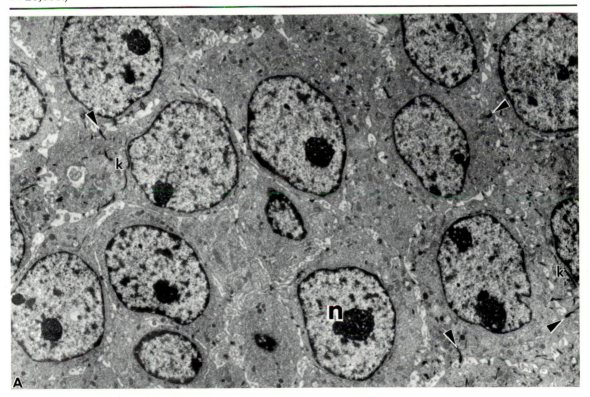

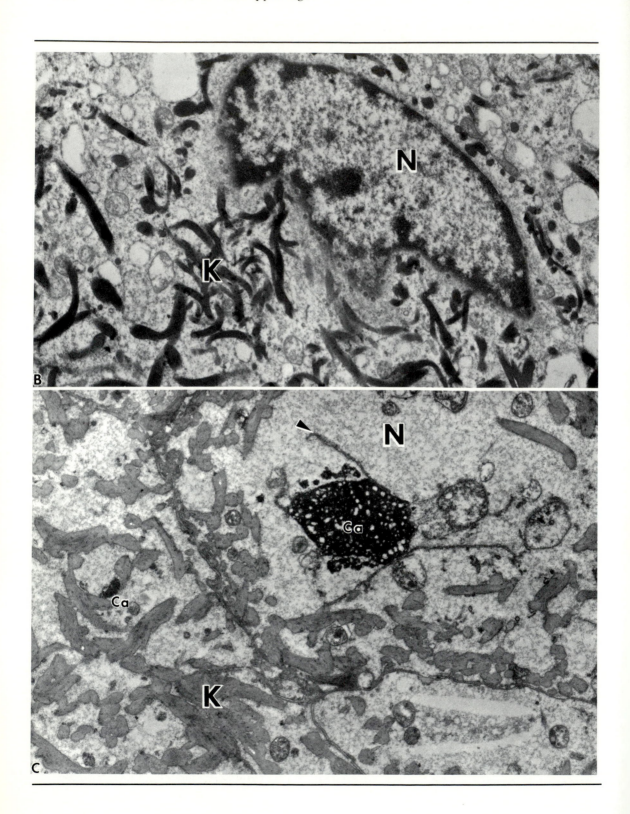

eration that apparently corresponds to or emerges from individual hair follicles (Fig. 1.4); (2) keratin cyst formation and foci of calcification that resemble
small trichoepithelioma; and (3) fibrous stroma that surround the epithelial
structures (Fig. 1.4).

Hair Follicle Nevus

Many well-differentiated but miniature hair follicles may be crowded in dome-
shaped or pedunculated lesions (Fig. 3.24). These follicles are surrounded with
a fibrous sheath.

Trichodiscomas and Multiple Fibrofolliculomas

The hair disc (Haarsheibe) is a specialized area of the skin field composed of
a hair, Merkel cells within the adjacent epidermis, and rich vascular component in the upper dermis. In trichodiscoma, a putative tumor of the hair disc,
numerous small dome-shaped papules are present, either disseminated[71] or
localized in one area[72] (Fig. 3.25A). Trichodiscomas may occur in association
with multiple fibrofolliculomas and acrochordons.[12,13] The patient with multiple fibrofolliculomas may also have a large connective tissue nevus but trichodiscomas has not been reported in association with connective tissue nevus.
If, however, multiple fibrofolliculomas coexist with trichodiscomas, it is difficult to differentiate the two lesions clinically.

Histology
Trichodiscoma is rather simple in appearance: dome-shaped fibrous tumor
fills the upper dermis under atrophic epidermis (Fig. 3.25). In most tumors
vascular components, elastic fibers, and some nerves are prominent but in
others only a richly mucinous fibrous tissue is found (Fig. 3.25). As in a
normal hair disc, a hair follicle may be present at one end of the papular
lesion.

   In fibrofolliculoma, the keratin-plugged, and often distorted hair follicle is
found in the center. A mantle of mucoid or fibrous stroma binds the periphery
of this central follicle. Thin epithelial cords emerge from the central follicle,
anastomose to each other, and form a net-like pattern (Fig. 3.26).

   Perifollicular fibroma is similar to fibrofolliculoma in histology but there
are no proliferative epithelial cords (Fig. 3.27). It represents de novo proliferation of the perifollicular connective tissue and not secondary fibrosis[73–75];
the fact that a congenital case was reported[74] supports this opinion.

Electron Microscopy
Two previous studies[13,14] and our own experience indicate that no Merkel
cells are present in the epidermis in trichodiscoma. Fibrous long-spacing (FLS)
collagen has been found in the mucinous connective tissue. The absence of

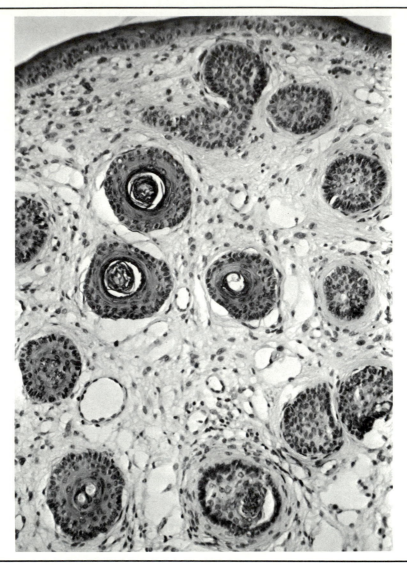

Figure 3.24
Hair follicle nevus. Many small hair follicles of vellus hair sizes are clustered. They are embedded in the fibrous and vascular stroma. (× 163.)

Figure 3.25
Trichodiscoma. In A a patient shows many small dome-shaped papules, 1 to 2 mm in diameter, on his lower trunk (arrowheads). The surface is smooth and flesh-colored. In B a scanning view of a typical dome-shaped papule is shown. There are fibrosis (F) as well as mucinosis (M) within the papule. In C the mucinous changes (M) are diffuse in the subepidermal region. The epidermis shows pressure atrophy. There are many clear keratinocytes (arrowheads) in the basal layer; these are neither melanocytes nor Merkel cells. In D fibrotic (F) rather than mucinous area is enlarged from different case. In E a focal mucinous degeneration caused a dissolution of dermal tissue to form a cavity (C). Hair follicle (H) is often associated with these papules (B and E). (B, × 10; C, × 100; D and E, × 163.)

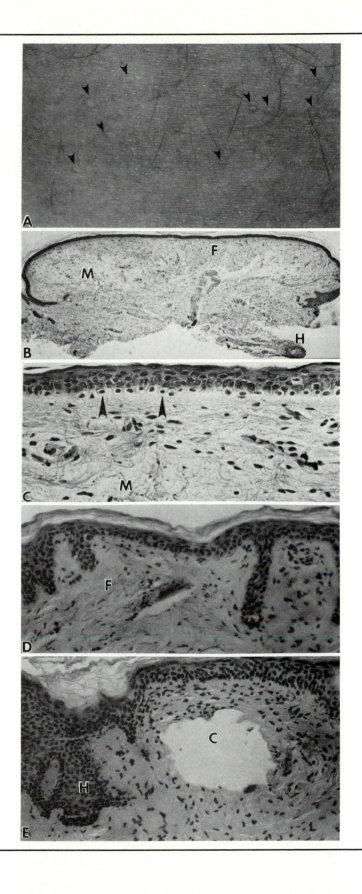

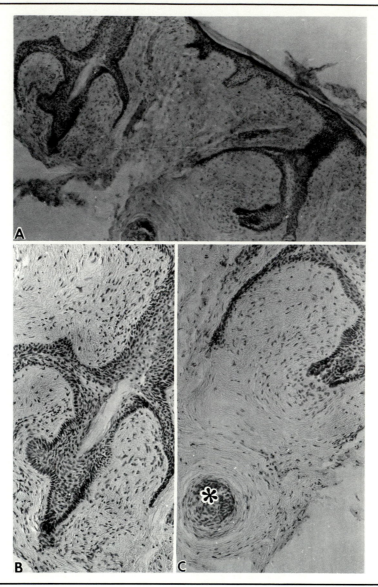

Figure 3.26
Fibrofolliculoma. In A, two proliferative follicular structures are surrounded with tightly bound fibrous tissues. In B and C, each follicular structure is enlarged. A hair bulb-like structure (*) is also seen. (A, × 130; B and C, × 163.)

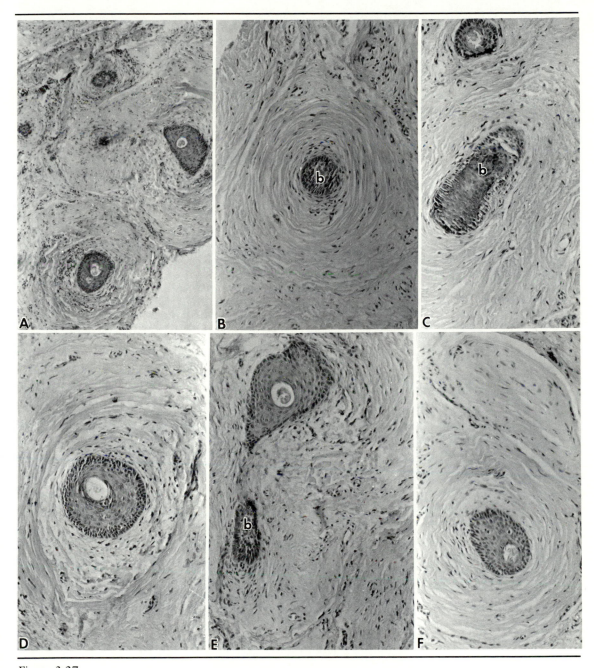

Figure 3.27
Perifollicular fibroma. In these pictures follicular structures, including hair bulb-like structures (b), are tightly bound by fibrous connective tissue. However, there are no proliferative features in these follicles. (A, × 65; B–F, × 163.)

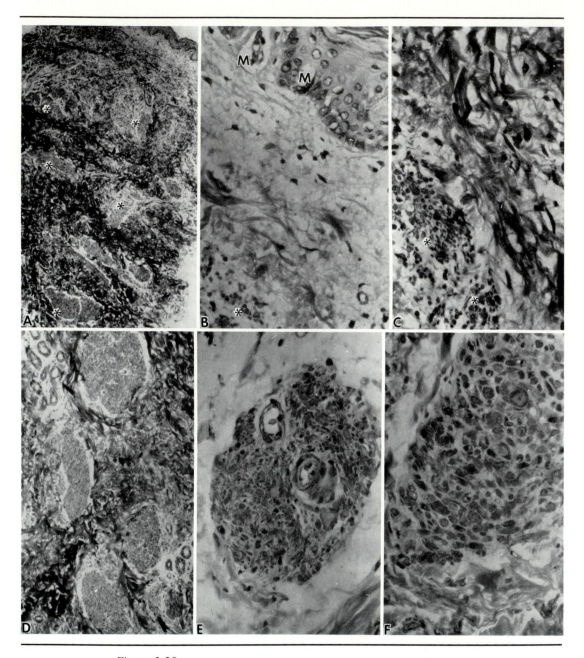

Figure 3.28
Arrector pili muscle hamartoma. In A, scattered islands of smooth muscle prolifera-
tion (*) are surrounded with dense collagen. In B, the epidermis covering the lesion
contains large vacuolated melanocytes (M); this area is hyperpigmented. Clinically,
this lesion was pigmented but no hair was seen. Loosely bundled small fibers (*) are
seen. In C, a superficial lesion is characterized by loosely bound, small fibers (*). In
D–F deep lesions are demonstrated; these are composed of tightly aggregated
smooth muscle fibers of strikingly variable sizes. In E, blood vessels are included in
the lesion but there is space between the tumor cells, indicating that vascular smooth
muscles are not participating. E and F—trichrome stain. (A, × 32; D, × 62; B, C,
E, and F, × 156.)

Merkel cells by electron microscopy seems to weaken the concept that trichodiscoma represents a hair disc tumor,[71] although one may argue that trichodiscoma represents a proliferation of only the fibrovascular components of the hair disc.[71]

Becker's Pigmented Hairy Nevus or Becker's Melanosis

This is a large pigmented patch with hypertrichosis that occurs most commonly over one shoulder or chest wall.[76] It is usually well-defined and shows a smooth, velvety surface and uniform hyperpigmentation. The onset is usually in the teens and hyperpigmentation always precedes hypertrichosis.[77] The hairs in the lesion are usually coarse terminal hairs. Vellus hairs may also be increased. In some lesions an increased number of irregularly arranged hypertrophic arrector pili muscles may be present and without particular relationship to the hair, although follicular papules or slight induration may occur.[78] After a vigorous rubbing the lesion becomes indurated due to contraction of the smooth muscles.[79] This so-called arrector pili muscle hamartoma may occur independently[79] or as a congenital lesion associated with Becker's melanosis[80,81] (Fig. 3.28).

REFERENCES

1. Mehregan AH. Pinkus' guide to dermatohistopathology. Norwalk CT: Appleton-Century-Crofts, 1986, 4th ed.
2. Mehregan AH. Infundibular tumors of the skin. J Cutan Pathol 1984;11:387–395.
3. Mehregan AH. Tumor of follicular infundibulum. Dermatologica 1971;142:177–183.
4. Winer LH. The dilated pore, a trichoepithelioma. J Invest Dermatol 1954;23:181–188.
5. Klövekorn G, Klövekorn W, Plewig G, Pinkus H. Riesenpore und haarscheidenakanthom. Klinische und histologische Diagnose. Hautarzt 1983;34:209–216.
6. Mehregan AH, Rahbari H. Benign epithelial tumors of the skin. III. Benign hair follicle tumors. Cutis 1977;19:595–599.
7. Mehregan AH, Brownstein MH. Pilar sheath acanthoma. Arch Dermatol 1978;114:1495–1497.
8. Bhawan J. Pilar sheath acanthoma: A new benign follicular tumor. J Cutan Pathol 1979;6:438–440.
9. Smolle J, Kerl M. Das "Pilar Sheath Acanthoma" ein gutartiges follikulares Hamartom. Dermatologica 1983;167:335–338.
10. Pinkus H, Sutton RL Jr. Trichofolliculoma. Arch Dermatol 1965;91:46–49.
11. Plewig G: Sebaceous trichofolliculoma. J Cutan Pathol 1980;7:394–403.
12. Birt AR, Hogg GR, Dube J. Hereditary multiple fibrofolliculomas with trichodiscomas and acrochordons. Arch Dermatol 1977;113:1674–1677.
13. Fujita WH, Barr RJ, Headley JL. Multiple fibrofolliculomas with trichodiscomas and acrochordons. Arch Dermatol 1981;117:32–35.
14. Weintraub R, Pinkus H. Multiple fibrofolliculomas (Birt-Hogg-Dube) associated with a large connective tissue nevus. J Cutan Pathol 1977;4:289–299.

15. Brownstein MH, Mehregan AH, Bikowski J, Lupulescu A, Patterson JC. The dermatopathology of Cowden's syndrome. Br J Dermatol 1979;100:667–673.
16. Brownstein MH, Shapiro L. The pilosebaceous tumors. Int J Dermatol 1977;16:340–352.
17. Starink TM, Hausman R. The cutaneous pathology of extrafacial lesions in Cowden's disease. J Cutan Pathol 1984;11:338–344.
18. Starink TM, Hausman R. The cutaneous pathology of facial lesions in Cowden's disease. J Cutan Pathol 1984;11:331–337.
19. Starink TM, Meijer CJLM, Brownstein MH. The cutaneous pathology of Cowden's disease: New findings. J Cutan Pathol 1985;12:83–93.
20. Mehregan AH. Inverted follicular keratosis. Arch Dermatol 1964;89:229–235.
21. Mehregan AH. Inverted follicular keratosis is a distinct follicular tumor. Am J Dermatopathol 1983;5:467–470.
22. Lever W, Schaumberg-Lever G. Histopathology of the skin. Philadelphia: JB Lippincott 1983, 6th ed., p 480.
23. Esterly NB, Fretzin DF, Pinkus H. Eruptive vellus hair cysts. Arch Dermatol 1977;113:500–503.
24. Stiefler RE, Bergfeld WF. Eruptive vellus hair cysts: An inherited disorder. J Am Acad Dermatol 1980;3:425–429.
25. Piepkorn MW, Clark L, Lombardi DL. A kindred with congenital vellus hair cysts. J Am Acad Dermatol 1981;5:661–665.
26. Kumakiri M, Takashima I, Iju M, Nogawa M, Miura Y. Eruptive vellus hair cysts: A facial variant. Am Acad Dermatol 1982;7:461–467.
27. Lee S, Kim JG. Eruptive vellus hair cyst. Arch Dermatol 1979;115:744–746.
28. Fritisch P, Wittels W. Ein Fall von bilateralem Naevus comedonicus. Hautarzt 1971;22:409–412.
29. Paige TN, Mandelson CG. Bilateral nevus comedonicus. Arch Dermatol 1967;96:172–175.
30. Wood MG, Thew MA: Nevus comedonicus. Arch Dermatol 1968;98:111–116.
31. Marsden RA, Fleming K, Dawber RPR. Comedo naevus of the palm. A sweat duct naevus? Br J Dermatol 1979;101:717–722.
32. Abell E, Read SI. Porokeratotic eccrine ostial and dermal duct nevus. Br J Dermatol 1980;103:435–441.
33. Barsky S, Doyle JA, Winkelmann RK. Nevus comedonicus with epidermolytic hyperkeratosis. Arch Dermatol 1971;117:86–88.
34. Plewig G, Christophers E. Nevoid follicular epidermolytic hyperkeratosis. Arch Dermatol 1975;111:223–226.
35. Nikolowski W. Tricho-Adenom. Arch Klin Exp Dermatol 1958;207:34–45.
36. Rahbari H, Mehregan A, Pinkus H. Trichoadenoma of Nikolowski. J Cutan Pathol 1977;4:90–98.
37. Egbert BM, Price NM, Sega RJ. Steatocystoma multiplex: Report of a florid case and a review. Arch Dermatol 1979;115:334–335.
38. Steatocystoma multiplex: A case presentation. Michigan Dermatological Society at Wayne State University, Nov. 7, 1984.
39. Brownstein MH. Steatocystoma simplex: A solitary steatocystoma. Arch Dermatol 1982;118:409–411.
40. Hashimoto K, Fisher BK, Lever WF. Steatocystoma multiplex. Hautarzt 1964;15:299–305.
41. Hashimoto K, Lever WF. Appendage tumors of the skin. Springfield, Ill.; Charles C. Thomas, 1968.
42. Pinkus H. "Sebaceous cysts" are trichilemmal cysts. Arch Dermatol 1969;99:544–555.

43. Leppard BJ, Sanderson KY, Wells RS. Hereditary trichilemmal cysts. Clin Exp Dermatol 1977;2:23–32.
44. Grayson S, Johnson-Winegar AG, Wintroub BU, Isseroff RR, Epstein EH, Elias PM. Lamellar body-enriched fractions from neonatal mice: Preparative techniques and partial characterization. J Invest Dermatol 1985;85:289–294.
45. Freinkel R, Traczyk TN. Lipid composition and acid hydrolase content of lamellar granules of fetal rat epidermis. J Invest Dermatol 1985;85:295–298.
46. Hashimoto K, Shibazaki S. Ultrastructural study on differentiation and function of hair. In: Toda K, Ishibashi Y, Hori Y, Morikawa F, eds., Biology and disease of the hair. Tokyo: University of Tokyo Press, 1976; pp 23–57.
47. Hashimoto K, Eto H, Matsumoto M, Hori K. Anti-keratin monoclonal antibodies: Production, specificities and applications. J Cutan Pathol 1983;10:529–539.
48. Pinkus H, Iwasaki T, Mishima Y. Outer root sheath keratinization in anagen and catagen of the mammalian hair follicle. A seventh distinct type of keratinization in the hair follicle: Trichilemmal keratinization. J Anat 1981;133:19–35.
49. Brownstein MH. Hybrid cyst: A combined epidermoid and trichilemmal cyst. J Am Acad Dermatol 1983;9:872–875.
50. Wilson-Jones E. Proliferating epidermoid cysts. Arch Dermatol 1966;94:11–19.
51. Dabska M. Giant hair matrix tumor. Cancer 1971;28:701–706.
52. Stranc MF, Bennett MH, Mehmed EP. Pilar tumour of the scalp developing in hereditary sebaceous cysts. Br J Plast Surg 1971;24:82–85.
53. Ploch PH, Muller HD. Pilartumor der Kopfhaut. Hautarzt 1979;30:84–88.
54. Yoshikawa K, Nakanishi A. A proliferating trichilemmal cyst on the back. J Dermatol (Tokyo) 1978;5:279–282.
55. Leppard BJ, Sanderson KV. The natural history of trichilemmal cysts. Br J Dermatol 1976;94:379–390.
56. Ziprkowski L, Schewach-Millet M. Multiple trichoepithelioma in a mother and two children. Dermatologica 1956;132:248–256.
57. Muller-Hess S, Delacretaz J. Trichoepitheliom mit Strukturen eines apokrinen Adenoms. Dermtologica 1973;146:170–176.
58. Brownstein MH, Shapiro L. Desmoplastic trichoepithelioma. Cancer 1977;40:2979–2986.
59. MacDonald DM, Wilson Jones E, Marks R. Sclerosing epithelial hamartoma. Clin Exp Dermatol 1977;2:153–160.
60. Headington JT. Tumors of the hair follicle. Am J Pathol 1976;85:480–514.
61. Headington JT. Selected pilar neoplasms: Appendage tumors with follicular differentiation. Course on adnexal neoplasms presented at the 21st Annual Meeting of the American Society of Dermatopathology. Chicago, Ill: 28 November 1983.
62. Chiaramonti A, Gilgor RS. Pilomatricoma associated with myotonic dystrophy. Arch Dermatol 1978;114:1363–1365.
63. Hashimoto K, Nelson RG, Lever WF. Calcifying epithelioma of Malherbe: Histochemical and electron microscopic studies. J Invest Dermatol 1966;46:391–408.
64. Brown AC, Crounse RG, Winkelmann RK. Generalized hair follicle hamartoma. Associated with alopecia, aminoaciduria and myasthenia gravis. Arch Dermatol 1969;99:478–493.
65. Ridley CM, Smith N. Generalized hair follicle hamartoma associated with alopecia and myasthenia gravis: Report of a second case. Clin Exp Dermatol 1982;6:283–289.
66. Carney RG. Linear unilateral basal cell nevus with comedones: Report of a case. Arch Dermatol 1952;65:471–476.
67. Anderson TE, Best PV. Linear basal cell nevus. Br J Dermatol 1962;74:20–23.

68. Bleiberg J, Brodkin RH. Linear unilateral basal cell nevus with comedones. Arch Dermatol 1969;100:187–190.
69. Kraus Z, Vortel V. Unilateral indolent basal cell nevus with comedones. Exp Med Sec XIV Derm Venereol 1961;51:121.
70. Mehregan AH, Baker S. Basaloid follicular hamartoma: Three cases with localized and systematized unilateral lesions. J Cutan Pathol 1985;12:55–65.
71. Pinkus H, Coskey R, Burgess GH. Trichodiscoma: A benign tumor related to the Haarscheibe (hair disk). J Invest Dermatol 1974;63:212–218.
72. Grosshans E, Dungler T, Hanau D. Le trichodiscome de Pinkus. Ann Dermatol Venereol 1981;108:837–846.
73. Zackheim HS, Pinkus H. Perifollicular fibromas. Arch Dermatol 1960;82:913–917.
74. Cramer HJ. Multiple perifollikulare Fibrome. Hautarzt 1968;19:228–229.
75. Freeman RG, Chernosky ME. Perifollicular fibroma. Arch Dermatol 1969;100:66–69.
76. Becker SW: Concurrent melanosis and hypertrichosis in distribution of nevus unius lateris. Arch Dermatol Syph 1949;60:155–160.
77. Gartmann H, Neuhas D, Tritsch H. Melanosis naeviformis. Z Hautkr 1968;43:973–984.
78. Urbanek RW, Johnson WC. Smooth muscle hamartoma associated with Becker's nevus. Arch Dermatol 1978;114:98–99.
79. Slifman NR, Harist TJ, Rhodes AR. Congenital arrector pili hamartoma: A case report and review of the spectrum of Becker's melanosis and pilar smooth-muscle hamartoma. Arch Dermatol 1985;121:1034–1037.
80. Plewig G, Schmoeckel C. Naevus musculi arrector pili. Hautarzt 1979;30:503–505.
81. Bonafé JL, Ghrenassia-Canal S, Vancina S. Naevus musculaire lisse. Ann Dermatol Venereol 1980;107:929–931.

4

Sebaceous Gland Tumors

The hair follicle originates from a column of germinative epithelium (hair germ) that descends at an angle from the epidermis to the dermis during the fourth month of fetal life. Sebaceous glands bud from the undersurface of the column. Since hair germs emerge from the basal layer of the epidermis, sebaceous glands share some characteristics of the epidermis such as keratinization of their duct walls. Germinative cells lining the periphery of the gland are identical to basal cells of the epidermis if one ignores early signs of sebum production. Sebaceous differentiation is obvious in all tumors of sebaceous gland origin except for very malignant varieties. Lipid stains are helpful in differentiating between clear cells arising from sebaceous gland and cells of eccrine or hair follicle origin, which contain glycogen rather than lipids. Ultrastructural demonstration of well-developed Golgi–smooth endoplasmic reticulum or lipid formation in these organelles help to differentiate sebaceous cells from other types of fat-containing cells such as lipidized histiocytes or lipocytes of fat tissue.

Sebaceous hyperplasia, a simple overgrowth of sebaceous gland without cytological abnormalities, may occur in four conditions: senile sebaceous hyperplasia, Fordyce spots, premature sebaceous gland hyperplasia, and organoid nevus.

Senile Sebaceous Hyperplasia

This small, yellowish papule may exhibit a central umbilication and, in rare cases, a hair. It occurs on sun-exposed skin where sebaceous glands are abundant, such as the forehead and cheeks. A common tumor of middle-aged or older white males, it clinically is often confused with basal cell epithelioma.

Histology

One large sebaceous gland with multiple clusters of sebaceous lobules usually surrounds a centrally located, dilated follicle pore (Fig. 4.1A). Generally one, and occasionally a few, layers of small basaloid germinative cells surround the periphery of each lobule (Fig. 4.1B). These very superficial glands are almost always in contact with the covering epidermis, which is atrophic from pressure (Fig. 4.1A); thus the yellowish color of the enlarged gland is transmitted to the surface.

Fernandez and Torres described four cases with linearly arranged papular lesions on the face in which hyperplastic sebaceous glands are found.[1] They called these lesions *linear* or *zoniform hyperplasia of sebaceous glands*. Their

Figure 4.1
Senile sebaceous gland hyperplasia. In A, a dilated pore (arrowhead) corresponds to a large follicular opening in which a hair has been compressed by an enlarged sebaceous gland (S₁) and has disappeared. Another gland (S₂) is apparently connected to the dilated follicle just above it and is situated very close to the atrophic epidermis. In B, single or double layers of basophilic or germinative cells surround the periphery of each lobule. Their maturation into clear sebocytes toward the center of the lobule proceeds in normal fashion. (A, × 65; B, × 163.)

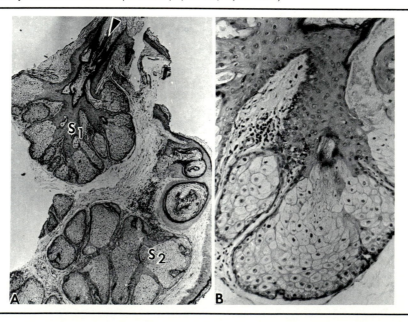

description of the lesions and the onset at puberty, however, suggest that these are a variant of nevus sebaceus. Blanchet-Bardon et al.[2] reported a 58-year-old white female with cutis verticis gyrata-like folding of forehead skin, with multiple greasy yellowish papules 1 to 2 mm in diameter, each of which had a central pore. Histologic examination revealed hyperplastic but nonproliferative sebaceous glands in each papule. After one month of therapy with 13-cis-retinoic acid, the lesions showed marked improvement, both clinically and histologically.

Fordyce's Spots (Granules or Condition)

Multiple small papules are clustered in the vermilion border of the lower lip or oral mucous membrane, particularly along the occlusal line. It is rather common among elderly individuals.

Histology
A small mature sebaceous gland is found in each papule. Although the duct leading to the mucosal surface may or may not be included in one section it usually is found in the serial sections. The histologic picture is essentially the same as senile sebaceous gland hyperplasia (Fig. 4.1).

Premature Sebaceous Gland Hyperplasia

This condition begins at puberty or in the twenties.[3–5] In one report it was familial.[3] Pits and lumps[4] consisting of 1- to 2-mm well-defined, yellow papules appear on the face in clusters, commonly on the chin.[5] Individual papules may show central umbilication. Because of its early onset, the large number of the lesions, and distribution on the chin rather than on the nose, this entity differs from rosacea or rhinophyma.

Histology
Histologic study reveals a mature sebaceous gland in the hyperplastic state and minimal infiltration by lymphocytes.

Nevus Sebaceus of Jadassohn or Organoid Nevus

Nevus sebaceus is the proper name for this lesion if one wishes to emphasize the fully developed stage of this nevoid lesion. However, there are early stages when the sebaceous component of the lesion is negligible. "Organoid nevus" would be a better term to cover the entire spectrum of growth involving the epidermis, the hair follicles, and the sebaceous and apocrine glands.[6] "Pilo-syringo-sebaceus-nevus"[7] is even more specific because it describes the entire contents of the lesion.

The lesion commonly manifests itself clinically at birth and in the infantile stage as a well-defined area of hair loss in which the skin is initially smooth or slightly verrucous (Fig. 4.2A). Discoloration is usually yellowish or dark brown. In adolescence the lesion becomes verrucous or peau d'orange-like. In the adult or late stage, it may be complicated by the development of various tumors and thus its clinical appearance changes accordingly.

The lesion usually appears alone, may be linear, and is almost always found on the head, neck, and face (Fig. 4.2B). In *neurocutaneous syndrome*[8-11] linear nevus sebaceous may be associated with epilepsy, mental retardation, and skeletal deformities.[12]

Histology

In the infantile stage the lesion generally reveals a slightly thickened epidermis, small hair follicles or hair germ-like epithelial nests, and an inconspicuous sebaceous gland. The apocrine glands are not yet recognizable (Fig. 4.3A). In adolescence a hyperkeratotic and acanthotic epidermis, hyperplastic sebaceous glands (Fig. 4.4A, B), and dilated apocrine glands are present. Hair follicles are not fully developed and usually remain at the hair germ stage (Fig. 4.3 B–F). In the third or adult stage, the acanthotic epidermis with hyperkeratosis, sebaceous gland hyperplasia, and apocrine gland proliferation continue. In addition, various types of adnexal tumors may develop within the nevoid malformation. These include basal cell epithelioma, trichilemmoma, syringocystadenoma papilliferum, sebaceous tumors (adenoma, epithelioma), apocrine tumors (nevus, adenoma, epithelioma), and others.[7]

In a recent study by Morioka[7] of 86 cases reviewed, the sebaceous glands, which were the major component of this tumor, were absent in 5.8%, normal in 25.5%, slightly proliferative in 38.3%, and markedly proliferative in 30.2%. The normal sebaceous glands are found more frequently from birth to 10 years of age but also in adolescence (14.7%) and among adult patients (16.1%). Absence of sebaceous gland hyperplasia and normal hair follicle development in an adult patient may justify a change in the diagnosis to a linear verrucous epidermal nevus.

The epidermal changes are also variable. According to the study by Morioka[7] the epidermis can be either acanthotic or nonacanthotic regardless of age. The acanthotic epidermis seems to possess characteristics of the outer root sheath of hair follicle; this feature can be rendered more apparent by stimulation such as stripping of the surface of the lesion.[7] Stripping with Scotch tape may induce marked acanthosis in an epidermis that looks normal; acanthotic cells thus induced are clear ones resembling those of trichilemmoma.[7]

Sebaceous Adenoma

This is a rare tumor of old age, the average age being over 60.[13] It is a solitary tumor except in cases with Torre's syndrome and measures less than 1 cm but may reach a size as large as 9 cm.[13] Clinically it is often misdiagnosed as basal cell epithelioma.[14] The predilection site is the face, particularly the nose

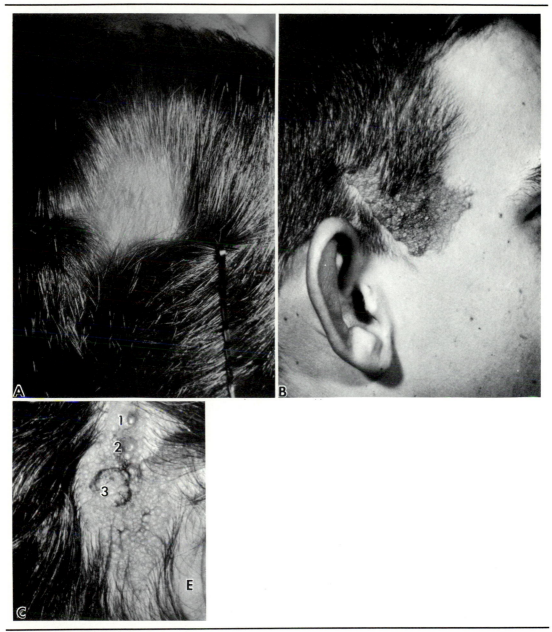

Figure 4.2
*Nevus sebaceus or organoid nevus. In A, alopecia in a child reveals slightly ele-
vated but rather smooth skin, representative of its early stage of nevus sebaceus. In
B, a pigmented verrucous lesion extends from the hairline to the preauricular area.
In the adult stage, shown here, the lesion is elevated, and the surface is verrucous. In
C, a pebbly-surfaced plaque behind the right ear (E) has developed three nodular
lesions (1, 2, 3). The top two nodules are bluish, and a biopsy revealed pigmented
basal cell epithelioma.*

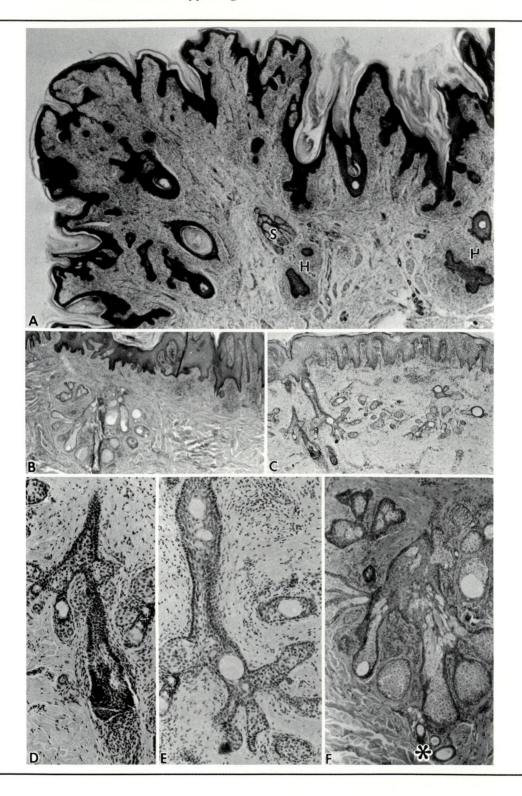

Figure 4.3
Nevus sebaceus or organoid nevus. In A, early stage development is limited to the formation of verrucous epidermis, a few abortive follicular structures (H), and a small sebaceous gland (S). In B–E, more advanced stages show development of hair germ-like structures. In F, the sebaceous glands are more mature. A few apocrine glands (*) are added. (A, × 100; B and C, × 65; D–F, × 130.)

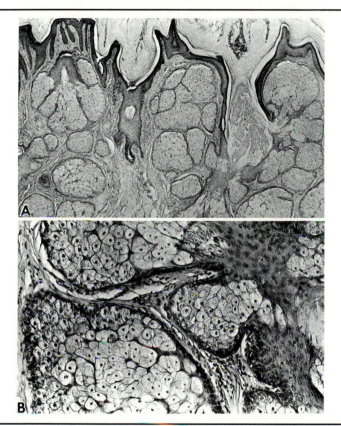

Figure 4.4
Nevus sebaceus or organoid nevus. In this lesion sebaceous gland hyperplasia predominates under the verrucous epidermis (A). Individual sebaceous glands are normal (B). (A, × 65; B, × 163.)

and cheek.[13,15,16] Occasionally sebaceous adenoma occurs in the mouth; it may originate from salivary gland or from Fordyce spots.[17,18] *Sebaceoma* is a term by Troy and Ackerman[19] who reported solitary papules or nodules on the face of mostly older white females. This entity seems to represent an admixture of a few conditions such as sebaceous adenoma, sebaceous epithelioma, and basal cell epithelioma with sebaceous differentiation. Some sebaceomas are similar to trichoepithelioma or cylindroma with sebaceous differentiation. These authors consider this entity to be a variant of sebaceous adenoma.

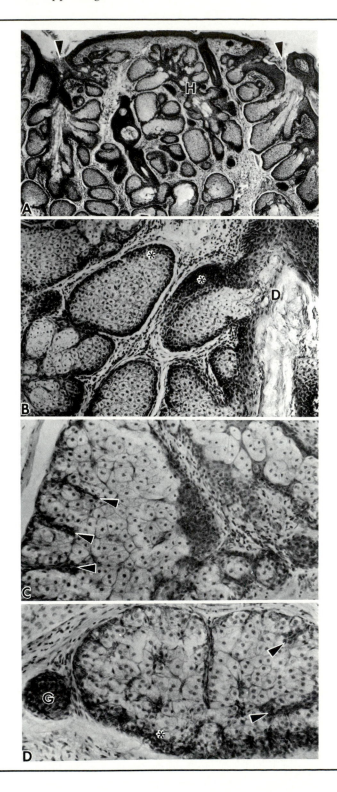

Histology

Sebaceous adenoma is well encapsulated by compressed collagen. A number of multilobulated sebaceous glands, which are mostly mature but often show retarded maturation, are present in the dermis (Fig. 4.5A). At the periphery of these lobules basophilic germinative cells are increased and often protrude into the lobules (Fig. 4.5B, C, D). Toward the ductal side of each lobule, differentiation of sebocytes is either complete and a small amount of holocrine degeneration occurs (Fig. 4.5B) or somewhat incomplete with small sebocytes without holocrine degeneration. The foci of such degeneration may enlarge and produce a large cyst. Sebaceous duct differentiation may occur in a form of squamous cell metaplasia. Mitosis and nuclear atypia are rare.

Sebaceous Epithelioma

Some authors prefer the term basal cell epithelioma with sebaceous differentiation.[13] In fact, clinical, histologic, and prognostic features of this tumor closely resemble basal cell epithelioma. Because some lesions are a yellowish color and most occur on the face there is some clinical resemblance to basal cell epithelioma. Ulceration and bleeding occur more frequently than in sebaceous adenoma. It is usually a solitary lesion less than 1 cm and is found on the sun-exposed skin of those middle-aged and older. It has been reported in the unusual location of the sole of the foot.[20] In rare instances it occurs multiply,[21] and multiple tumors may develop over a period of many years.[22] Sebaceous epithelioma may be found in nevus sebaceus of Jadassohn[7] and in Torre's syndrome.[23]

Histology

In contrast to sebaceous adenoma in which sebaceous cells predominate and basaloid or germinative cells are in the minority, sebaceous epithelioma shows just the opposite; a small number of sebocytes are scattered among a predominant basaloid tumor cell population (Fig. 4.6). The lobular architecture of normal sebaceous glands is often lost but cellular atypia and invasive features are minimal.

Sebaceous differentiation of basal cell epithelioma can occur in all subtypes

Figure 4.5

Sebaceous adenoma. In A, a large number of sebaceous glands are present, some which are connected to hair canal-like invaginations (arrowheads) or follicular structures (H). In B, including holocrine degeneration of sebocytes into the duct (D), individual sebaceous glands are normal except for some increase in germinative cells at the periphery (*). In C, these germinative cells invaginate into the lobule (arrowheads). In D, in addition to a thick germinative layer (*) which shows invaginations (arrowheads), a solid mass of germinative cells (G) is present. Mature sebocytes appear normal, and mitoses or cell atypia are absent. (A, × 52; B, × 130; C and D, × 163.)

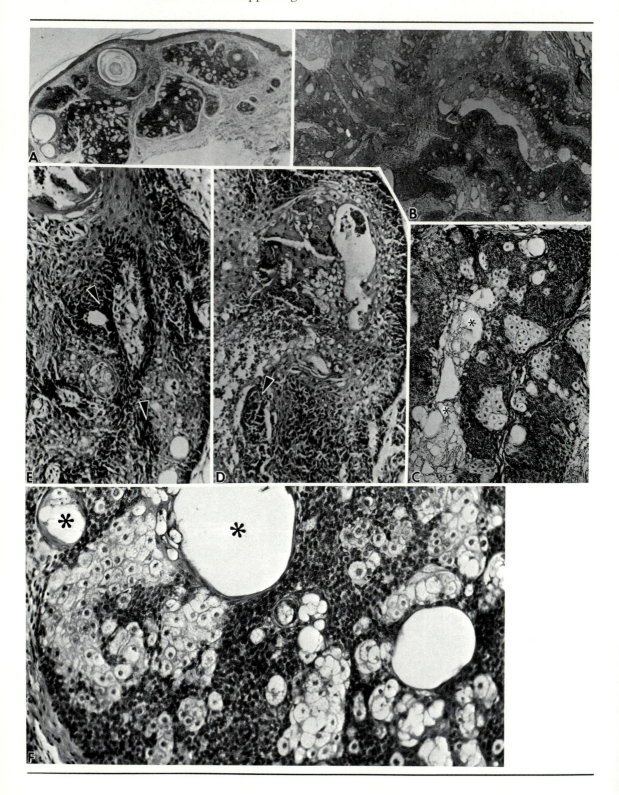

Figure 4.6
Sebaceous epithelioma. In A *and* B *the lesion looks like a keratotic or cystic basal cell epithelioma. In* C *and* F *the tumor is made primarily of germinative cells, and sebaceous cells tend to degenerate and form cystic spaces (*). In* D *and* E *the organization of tumor cells into gland is not distinct, although a thick band of hyperchromatic germinative cells (arrowheads) rim the periphery. (A,* × *22; B,* × *52; C,* × *65; D and E,* × *163; F,* × *200.) (Fig. 4.6C courtesy of Kan Niizuma, M.D. Fig. 4.6F courtesy of Martin C. Mihm, Jr., M.D.)*

including cystic basal cell epithelioma; thus it is sometimes difficult to separate this tumor from sebaceous epithelioma. It is our belief that genuine sebaceous epitheliomas do exist and that they are clinically and histologically more proliferative than are sebaceous adenoma but less malignant than sebaceous carcinoma. In Torre's syndrome this wide spectrum of sebaceous tumor differentiation and dedifferentiation is exhibited in the same patient who may or may not have basal cell epithelioma.[24] Electron microscopic examination by Niizuma revealed an ultrastructurally traceable maturation sequence—from immature cells to mature sebocytes through transitional cells.[25] These cells were richly equipped with lipid-producing organelles (Fig. 4.7),[25] a feature never observed in lipid degeneration of basal cell epithelioma. The complete absence of melanocytes is also evidence against the basal cell epithelioma origin of sebaceous epithelioma.

Sebaceous Carcinoma

Carcinoma of the sebaceous gland is rare. The eyelid is the most common site and tumors on this location are much more aggressive and metastasizing than those found on other sites. Meibomian glands of the tarsus and the Zeis gland are located at the lid margin of the eyelid as are the glands of the pilosebaceous unit; the increased number of glands may explain the increased frequency of malignancies. According to three large series,[26–28] the upper eyelid of women in their mid-sixties is the most common site. They are usually a solitary, deep-seated, and asymptomatic[26–28] mass and are often treated as a chalazion or blepharoconjunctivitis. Radiation therapy may predispose the skin for the tumor development.[29,30]

Occular sebaceous carcinomas are invasive. Metastasis usually occurs first to the regional lymph nodes such as the preauricular, submaxillary, and/or cervical ones. It may extend also to facial bones and metastasis to the viscera[5,31] may occur.

It is extremely rare for sebaceous carcinoma to be found anywhere but on the eyelid. When it does it is usually found as a solitary, pinkish red nodule of the head and neck region[13] that measures about 1 to 4 cm, only rarely is it larger (8 cm).[32] It is frequently ulcerated and may mimic a cyst, rhinophyma, or leukoplakia.[13] As it does on the eyelid, radiation therapy may predispose the skin to develop this malignant tumor.[33,34]

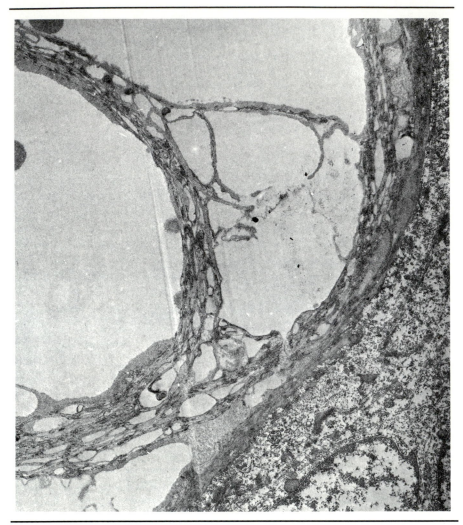

Figure 4.7
Sebaceous epithelioma. When sebaceous differentiation of a tumor cell occurs a stack of parallel layers of smooth-surfaced endoplasmic reticulum produces a lipid substance. These lamellar structures eventually shed into the vacuole as they would in normal sebaceous cells. (× 9,000.)

Histology

Sebaceous carcinoma exhibits all the histologic markers of malignancy. Large cells with hyperchromatic nuclei and mitotic figures are observed (Fig. 4.8B, C). Sebaceous cells are scattered but many of them may contain eosinophilic cytoplasm instead of the typical lipid droplets. Glandular architecture may be completely lost and unless a careful search is made, the sebaceous nature of the tumor may not be detected (Fig. 4.6A). Tumor masses invade the dermis and an inflammatory cell reaction surrounds them. Epidermal involvement may resemble Paget's disease.

Pathology

The tumor is an invasive one and can easily pass through the superficial striated muscle layer.[5] Once beyond this barrier the tumor can easily grow and metastasize in the loose tissue. These tumor cells tend to form lobules or show the tendency to aggregate. In very invasive tumors individual cells may invade the stroma. Large basophilic cells may contain bubbly cytoplasm but only a small percentage of tumor cells fully mature into sebaceous cells. The cytologic features of malignant cells are obvious, such as nuclear pleomorphism and hyperchromatism, frequent and bizarre mitosis, and cellular atypia.[5] In the eyelid lesion there is pagetoid infiltration of the epidermis and/or conjunctival epithelium.[5] These are large clear cells or vacuolated cells with a large nucleus and prominent nucleoli. In contrast to Paget cells, they stain positive for fat and negative for acid mucopolysaccharide.[27]

Tumors other than on the eyelid show essentially the same histologic features. They may deeply invade the dermis and metastasize widely despite good sebaceous differentiation of the tumor cells.[32]

Muir-Torre's Syndrome

This syndrome is often referred to as Torre's syndrome[35] but the first report was made by Muir et al.[36] and, therefore, is more appropriately termed the Muir-Torre syndrome. Since that initial report a total of 26 cases have been reported in the world literature.[23] The disease does not follow any established mode of inheritance but many cases exist in which a proband's family members had either intestinal carcinoma or sebaceous tumors.[23,24] Family members of those with autosomal dominant *cancer family syndrome,* a syndrome closely related to Muir-Torre syndrome,[35] often exhibit sebaceous tumors. Its onset ranges widely through adulthood. Multiple sebaceous tumors usually occur on the face and head (Fig. 4.9) and primary visceral carcinomas may be found. Sebaceous tumors range from sebaceous adenoma to sebaceous carcinoma and develop over many years. Nonsebaceous tumors include basal cell epithelioma, squamous cell carcinoma, and in particular, keratoacanthoma singly, multiply, or in combination. Visceral tumors are usually multiple and are often adenocarcinomas of the digestive tract, particularly of the colon.[23] Carcinoma of the larynx, bronchus, genitourinary tract and endometrium have been reported. Colorectal polyps are common. Although visceral tumors may precede the skin tumors in some cases, the opposite is also true and thus skin signs are important.[24]

Histopathology

Individual sebaceous tumors are indistinguishable from those that occur singly (Figs. 4.5, 4.6, and 4.8). Basal cell epithelioma and keratoacanthoma often exhibit sebaceous differentiation. Sebaceous carcinomas, though histologically malignant, seldom metastasize. In this syndrome visceral carcinomas behave rather benignly; with rare exceptions, they remain localized and do not metastasize.[13]

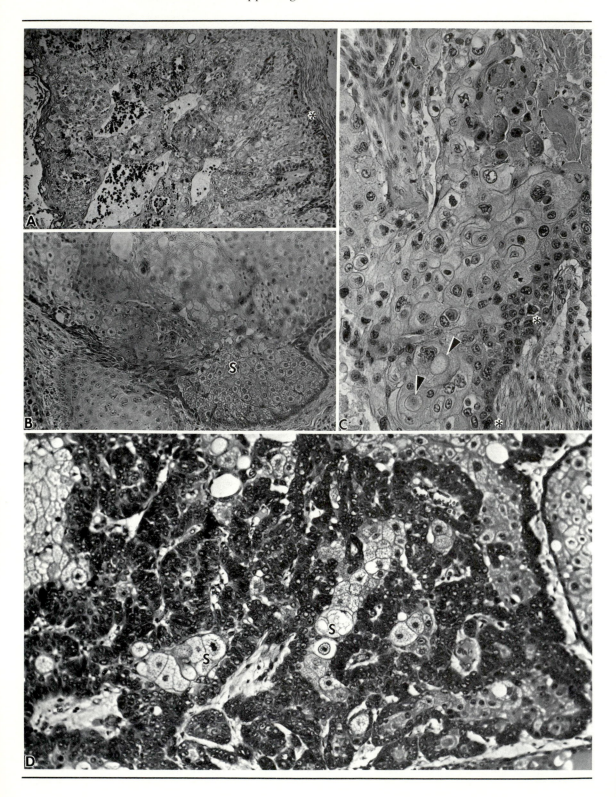

Figure 4.8
Sebaceous carcinoma. In A, irregular strands of epithelial tumor can barely be recognized as "sebaceous" because of some clear cells and peripheral germinative cells (*). In B, nuclear atypia is seen in irregularly sized sebocytes. A normal sebaceous gland (S) is attached. In C, large eosinophilic cells exhibiting nuclear hyperchromasia and atypia could be identified to be of sebaceous gland origin because of the few lipid droplets seen in large cells (arrowheads) and the peripheral germinative cells that also show atypia (*). In D, large tumor cells form anastomosing cords and strands. Irregular in shape and size but mature (foamy) sebocytes (S) intermingle with hyperchromatic malignant cells. (A, × 65; B and D, × 163; C, × 200.) (Fig. 4.7D courtesy of Martin C. Mihm, Jr., M.D.)

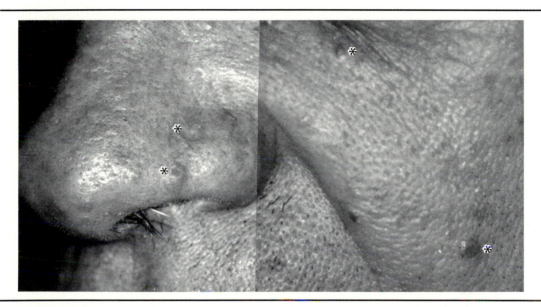

Figure 4.9
Muir-Torre's syndrome. The multiple facial tumors are sebaceous adenomas and epitheliomas. Clinically, these individual lesions are similar to senile sebaceous gland hyperplasia.

REFERENCES

1. Fernandez N, Torres A. Hyperplasia of sebaceous glands in a linear pattern of papules: Report of four cases. Am J Dermatopathol 1984;6:237–243.
2. Blanchet-Barden C, Servant JM, Bao LeTaun, Puissant A. Hyperplasie sébacée acquise a type de cutis verticis gyrata sensible au 13-Cis-Retinoid. Ann Derm Venereol 1982;109:749–750.
3. Dupre A, Bonafé JL, Lamon R. Functional familial sebaceous hyperplasia of the face. Clin Exp Dermatol 1980;5:203–207.
4. DeVillez RL, Roberts JC. Premature sebaceous gland hyperplasia. J Am Acad Dermatol 1982;6:933–935.

5. Prioleau PG, Santa Cruz DJ. Sebaceous gland neoplasia. J Cutan Pathol 1984; 11:396–414.

6. Mehregan AH, Pinkus H. Life history of organoid nevi: Special reference to nevus sebaceus of Jadassohn. Arch Dermatol 1965;91:574–588.

7. Morioka S. The natural history of nevus sebaceus. J Cutan Pathol 1985;12:200–213.

8. Schimmelpenning GW. Klinischer Beitrag zur Symptomatologie der Phakomatosen. Fortschr Roentgenstr 1957;87:716–720.

9. Feuerstein R, Mims L. Linear nevus sebaceus with convulsions and mental retardation. Am J Dis Child 1962;104:675–679.

10. Marden PM, Venters HD. A new neurocutaneous syndrome. Am J Dis Child 1966;112:79–81.

11. Wauschkuhn J, Rohde B. Systematisierte Talgdrüs en-, Pigment-, und epitheliale Naevi mit neurologischer Symptomatik; Feuerstein-Mimssches neuroektodermales Syndrom. Hautarzt 1971;22:10–13.

12. Hornstein OP, Knickenberg M. Zur Kenntnis des Schimmelpenning-Feuerstein-Mims-Syndroms. Arch Dermatol Forsch 1974;250:35–50.

13. Rulon DB, Helwig EB. Cutaneous sebaceous neoplasms. Cancer 1974;33:82–102.

14. Warren S, Warvi WN. Tumors of sebaceous glands. Am J Pathol 1943;19:441–460.

15. Brownstein MH, Shapiro L. The pilosebaceous tumors. Int J Dermatol 1977; 16:340–352.

16. Mehregan AH, Rahbari H. Benign epithelial tumors of the skin. II. Benign sebaceous tumors. Cutis 1977;19:317–320.

17. Epker BN, Henny FA. Intra-oral sebaceous gland adenoma. Cancer 1971;27:987–989.

18. Miller AS, McCrea MW. Sebaceous gland adenoma of the buccal mucosa: Report of a case. J Oral Surg 1968;26:593–595.

19. Troy JL, Ackerman AB. Sebaceoma: A distinctive benign neoplasm of adnexal epithelioma differentiating toward sebaceous cells. Am J Dermatopathol 1984;6:7–13.

20. Raab W: Talgdrüsenepitheliom. Arch Klin Exp Dermatol 1963;216:325–333.

21. Lasser A, Carter DM. Multiple basal cell epitheliomas with sebaceous differentiation. Arch Dermatol 1973;107:91–93.

22. Rothko K, Farmer ER, Zeligman I. Superficial epitheliomas with sebaceous differentiation. Arch Dermatol 1980;116:329–331.

23. Alessi E, Brambilla L, Luporini G, Mosga L, Bevilacqua G. Multiple sebaceous tumors and carcinomas of the colon: Torre syndrome. Cancer 1985;55:2566–2574.

24. Housholder MS, Zeligman I. Sebaceous neoplasms associated with visceral carcinomas. Arch Dermatol 1980;116:61–64.

25. Niizuma K. An electron microscopic study of sebaceous epithelioma: A case report with two new observations on lipid droplet formation. Dermatologica 1977; 154:98–106.

26. Bingkuan N, Chuo G. Pathologic classification of meibomian gland carcinomas of eyelids: Clinical and pathologic study of 156 cases. Chinese Med J (Peking) 1979;92:671–676.

27. Rao NA, Hidayat AA, McLean IW, Zimmerman LE. Sebaceous carcinomas of the ocula adnexa: A clinicopathologic study of 104 cases, with five-year follow-up data. Hum Pathol 1982;13:113–122.

28. Ni C, Kuo PK. Meibomian gland carcinoma: A clinicopathological study of 156 cases with long-period follow-up of 100 cases. Jap J Ophthalmol 1979;23:388–401.

29. Lemos LB, Santa Cruz DJ, Baba N. Sebaceous carcinoma of the eyelid following radiation therapy. Am J Surg Pathol 1978;2:305–321.
30. Schlernitzauer DA, Font RL. Sebaceous gland carcinoma of the eyelid. Arch Ophthalmol 1976;94:1523–1525.
31. Boniuk M, Zimmerman LE. Sebaceous carcinoma of the eyelid, eyebrow, carbuncle and orbit. Trans Am Acad Ophthalmol Otolaryngol 1968;72:619–642.
32. King DT, Hirose FM, Gurevitch AW. Sebaceous carcinoma of the skin with visceral metastases. Arch Dermatol 1979;115:862–863.
33. Justi RA. Sebaceous carcinoma: Report of case developing in area of radiodermatitis. Arch Dermatol 1958;77:195–200.
34. Urban FH, Winkelmann RK. Sebaceous malignancy. Arch Dermatol 1961;84:63–72.
35. Lynch HT, Lynch PM, Pester J, Fusaro RM. The cancer family syndrome: Rare cutaneous phenotypic linkage of Torre's syndrome. Arch Intern Med 1981;141:607–611.
36. Muir EG, Yates Bell AJ, Barlow KA. Multiple primary carcinomata of the colon, duodenum, and larynx associated with keratoacanthomata of the face. Br J Surg 1967;54:191.

5

Apocrine Tumors

The criteria for apocrine differentiation include the histologic observation of tall columnar epithelium with decapitation secretion; ultrastructural demonstration of the above and of large dense granules and/or mitochondria-derived light granules; and histochemical identification of lysosomal enzymes such as acid phosphatase and β-glucuronidase, and PAS-positive, diastase-resistant granules, iron-positive granules, and lipofuscin (Table 1.3). Specific monoclonal antibodies that react to only the apocrine gland have yet to be developed. Immunohistochemically, carcinoembryonic antigen (CEA) is present but is also found in eccrine structures and in their tumors (Table 1.5). Gross cystic disease fluid protein (GCDFP-15) of the breast was recently proposed as an apocrine marker[1,2] (Table 1.5).

The apocrine gland emerges from the hair germ just above the sebaceous gland anlage and, like sebaceous gland, attains full maturity in utero under maternal androgenic influence. Shortly after birth it undergoes atrophy as does the sebaceous gland and remains inactive until puberty. Thus, tumors of the apocrine gland are rare before puberty except for an occasional nevoid growth, such as those associated with nevus sebaceus (organoid nevus).[3] The short apocrine duct opens into the hair follicle. Although the intrafollicular portion resembles the embryonic acrosyringium of eccrine duct because there are some lysosomes, there is no tumor of this segment which corresponds to eccrine poroma. In the strict sense apocrine duct tumor does not even exist because apocrine hidrocystoma (or cystadenoma), unlike eccrine hidrocystoma, has myoepithelial cells, a hallmark of secretory differentiation. Only ductal tumors due to dilatation or retention are found in modified apocrine gland, that is, in Moll's glands. Thus, most of the apocrine tumors originate from or differentiate toward secretory segment. In this chapter those "definite apocrine tumors" with relatively simple structural organization are described first, and then those generally considered "probable apocrine tumors" are discussed as a group (Table 1.1).

Apocrine Nevus

Pure apocrine nevi are very rare. Reported lesions have occurred in the scalp,[4] axillae,[5] and in the sternal region,[6] and range from a solitary small nodule to multiple firm papules. Normal or slightly adenocystic apocrine glands are often found underlying the lesions of nevus sebaceus (organoid nevus) and syringocystadenoma papilliferum.

Histology

Apocrine glands are all mature and are only abnormal in number. Situated in the lower portion of the reticular dermis and subcutaneous tissue (Fig. 5.1), the tumor is mainly composed of secretory glands that may be partly secretory and partly atrophic and dilated. Ducts are also present but apparently they are not all connected to the hair follicles.

Apocrine Hidrocystoma or Apocrine Cystadenoma

This is almost always a solitary nodular cystic lesion commonly found on the face, head, neck, and upper torso. It is 3 to 15 mm in size[7] and often bluish black in color; therefore the clinician may consider blue nevus or malignant melanoma. Although extremely rare, Kruse et al.[8] reported a case with 40 lesions. It is found equally in men and women, and the average age is 55 years.[9] Lesions that have been reported on the penis[10,11] would be better regarded as median raphe cyst.[12] Apocrine cystadenoma may be associated with nevus sebaceus. Some of the dilated cystadenomas of chondroid syringoma show tall columnar luminal cells and decapitation secretion, and may resemble apocrine cystadenoma[13] (Fig. 2.27A).

Histology

In a small tumor the single cystic space is lined by two layers of wall cells; the inner layer consists of tall columnar cells revealing decapitation secretion in the eosinophilic apical portion, and the outer layer is made up of cuboidal or elongated myoepithelial cells, depending upon the angle of sectioning (Figs. 5.2E and 5.3). Along the periphery of the cyst a PAS-positive basement mem-

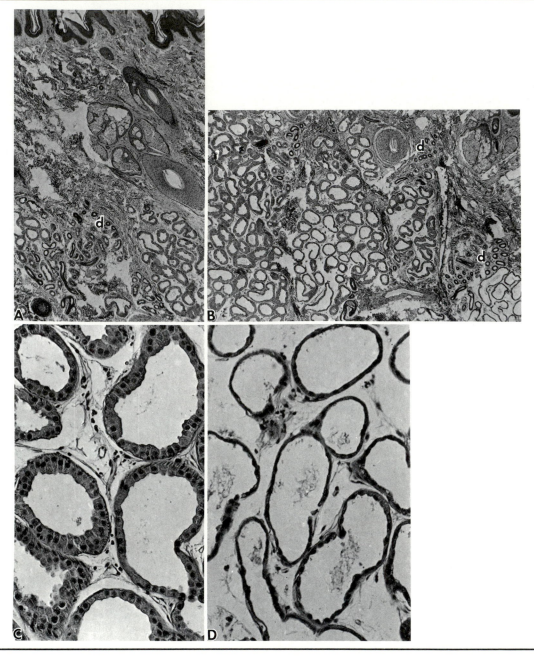

Figure 5.1
Apocrine nevus. In A and B, a large number of apocrine glands are found in the lower dermis. There are ducts (d) from these secretory segments but no openings, either to the epidermis or to the hair follicle. In C, these glands are slightly dilated but essentially normal in morphology. In D, secretory cells are flat and atrophic; this may represent postsecretory stages or pressure atrophy due to secretion products in occluded glands (A and B, × 52; C and D, × 163.)

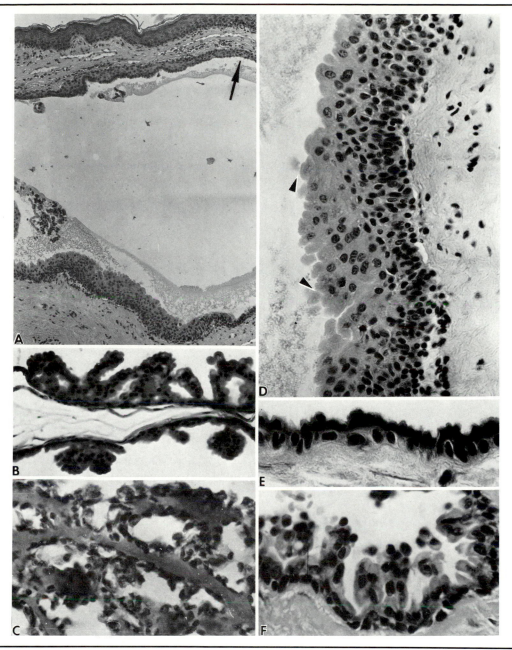

Figure 5.2
*Apocrine hidrocystoma or apocrine cystadenoma. Cystic spaces are lined by a wall
of two to several cell layers and contain cellular debris (A). At high magnification
the cyst wall is composed of columnar or cylindrical luminal cells and round, cuboidal, or rectangular basal cells (D, E, and F). The tip of the luminal cells shows
tearing-off or decapitation secretion (arrowheads in D). The wall may produce papillary projections (C) or tufts of overgrown luminal cells (B and F). In some cysts the
wall forms thin trabecular meshes that project into the lumen (C). The luminal wall
near the epidermis is flat and epidermoid (arrow in A). (A, × 65; B, × 149; C and
D, × 186; E and F, × 484.) (Fig. 5.2B courtesy of Martin C. Mihm, Jr., M.D.)*

brane can be demonstrated. In a large tumor the cyst wall protrudes into the lumen in multiple papillated or folded structures (Fig. 5.2C, F). Focal proliferation of the luminal cells in cluster or mushroom-like protrusions may be present (Fig. 5.2B). Near the epidermis the cystic structures are lined with a layer of flattened ductal epithelium[7] (Fig. 5.2A). In contrast to eccrine hidrocystoma, in which there is acute or chronic dilatation of the eccrine dermal duct, apocrine hidrocystoma is a proliferative adenoma of the apocrine secretory segment; thus it is an actively growing tumor, evidenced by papillary growth. In this sense, apocrine "cystadenoma" seems to be a better name, particularly for those large tumors with thick, folded papilliferous projections of the wall cells.

Histochemistry

PAS-positive, diastase-resistant secretory granules, probably lysosomal in nature, are found in the secretory cells. Eccrine-specific antigens as detectable with EKH5 and EKH6 are negative in most tumors[14] but positive in some, suggesting that there are "eccrine cystadenoma" among the apocrine cystadenomas determined histologically. This situation may be repeated in the classification of the tubular apocrine adenoma, which some authors call papillary eccrine adenoma (see below). The bluish black color is seen in one-third to half of apocrine hidrocystomas. The substance responsible for this color is not certain. Only occasionally the cyst contents are brownish and, therefore, the color should come from epithelial cells or surrounding connective tissue. The bluish black color may be due to lipofuscin,[15] hemosiderin,[16] or melanin,[17] (Fig. 5.3B) among other things. The Tyndall effect, analogous to that seen in the blue dome cyst of fibrocystic breast disease, has also been suggested.[17]

Electron Microscopy

The secretory cells that line the cystic space show typical decapitation secretion (Fig. 5.4), large dense granules of apocrine type, and annulate lamellae that are seen only in apocrine secretory cells.[16,18] The basally located myoepithelial cells are mature cells full of fibers (Fig. 5.3A). Thus, ultrastructurally, this tumor is a mature apocrine adenoma.

Figure 5.3
Apocrine hidrocystoma or apocrine cystadenoma. In A, a two-layer construction of the wall consists of myoepithelial cells (M) on the basal lamina (BL) and columnar secretory cells with long villi (V) lining the lumen. In B, melanin-like dense granules (m) are seen in a luminal cell with long luminal villi (V). One large aggregate of dense granules (M) is enlarged in the inset. (A, × 15,000; B, × 25,000; inset of B × 75,000.)

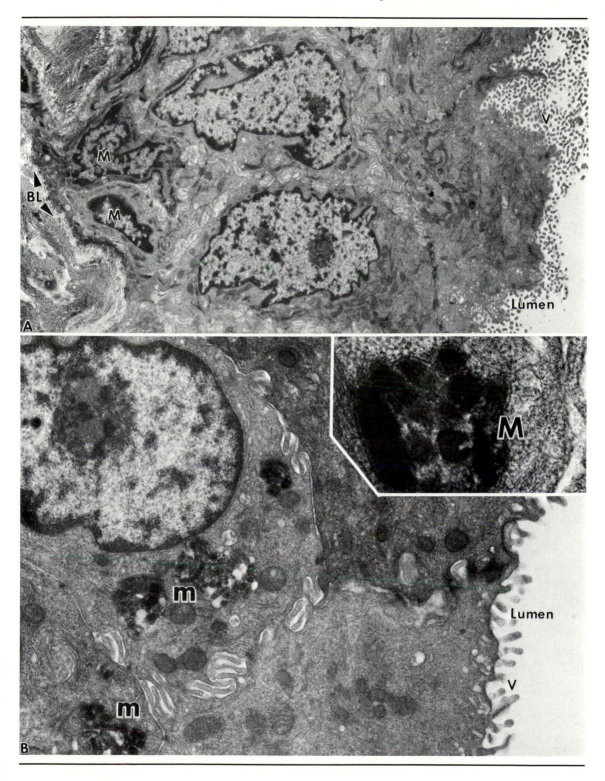

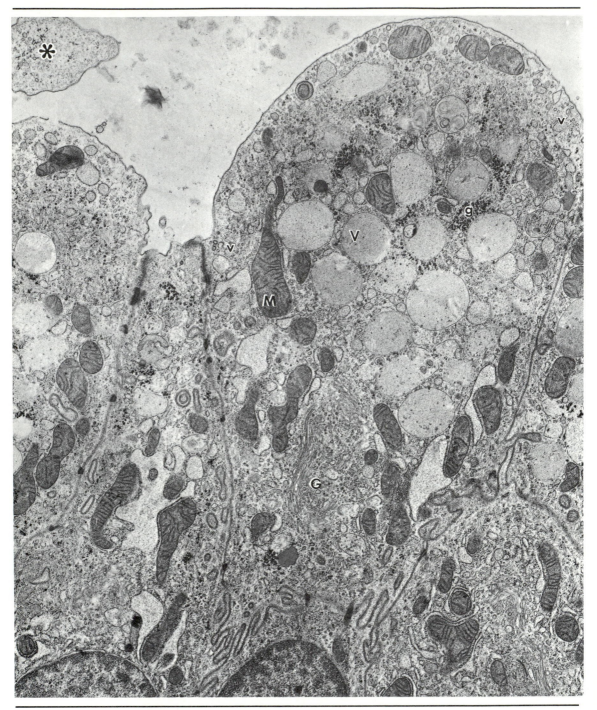

Figure 5.4
Apocrine hidrocystoma or apocrine cystadenoma. A typical secretory cell on the right shows apical swelling and contains many vacuoles (V), vesicles (v), mitochondria (M), some glycogen (g) and a Golgi apparatus (G); it is ready for decapitation secretion. The cell on the left has apparently lost apical cytoplasm; it is at a post-secretion stage. A part of segregated cytoplasm is still seen in the lumen (*). (× 8,000.)

Moll's Gland Cyst

On the eyelids, particularly on the inner or outer canthus of the palpebral border of the lower eyelid, a semitransparent cyst occurs (Fig. 5.5A, B). Moll's gland, a modified apocrine gland, empties its secretion into the eyelash follicle. Although generally solitary it is sometimes multiple. They may be less than a few millimeters or large enough to obstruct vision. The cyst may persist for many years without rupturing.

Histology

Most of these eyelid cysts are histologically similar to apocrine hidrocystoma (Fig. 5.5) with the exception that the basal cells surrounding the periphery of the cyst are not myoepithelial cells. The luminal cells are mostly ductal cells with short numerous villi and a periluminal band of tonofilaments. Some secretory cells with electron-light granules or numerous vacuoles and vesicles may be seen (Fig. 5.5G). Many luminal cells undergo partial keratinization; thus, keratohyalin granules are commonly found (Fig. 5.5F). Completely keratinized cells are rare; however, in some lesions the luminal spaces are filled with keratin (Fig. 5.5D, E, F). In some cysts goblet-like cells (Fig. 5D, E) similar to those of palpebral conjunctiva may be present. However, electron microscopy reveals that these cells are filled with fibrous aggregates, perhaps degenerated keratin filaments (Fig. 5.6), which may be discharged into the lumen; the keratinous debris seen in the cyst may in part derive from these cells (Fig. 5.5D, E) and also from the keratinizing wall cells (Fig. 5.5F).

Tubular Apocrine Adenoma, Apocrine Adenoma, and Apocrine Fibroadenoma

These are all extremely rare tumors. Tubular apocrine adenoma may occur in association with nevus sebaceus of the scalp[19–21] and resembles, or is identical to, papillary eccrine adenoma.[22] Apocrine adenoma occurs in both sexes and may be found anywhere; however, apocrine areas such as the perianal region[23] and the axilla[24] are favored. Apocrine fibroadenoma occurs in the perianal and vulvar regions,[25,26] and may be multiple.[26] Clinically, these tumors are uncharacteristic in that they may be nodular or pedunculated. *Ceruminous adenoma* of the external auditory canal's ceruminous gland is histologically identical to cutaneous apocrine adenoma, although so-called *ceruminomas* refer to miscellaneous glandular and adenomatous tumors.

Histology

Apocrine adenoma shows more solid cellular (epithelial) component (Fig. 5.7D, E) than the dilated cystic structures like those seen in apocrine cystadenoma (Fig. 5.7A, B, C). However, the proportion of cystic and epitheliomatous elements varies from one lesion to another[29] (Fig. 5.7C). In tubular apocrine adenoma, dermal and subcutaneous lobulated tumor masses are composed of dilated and branching tubular adenomatous structures (Fig. 5.7F, G). One or

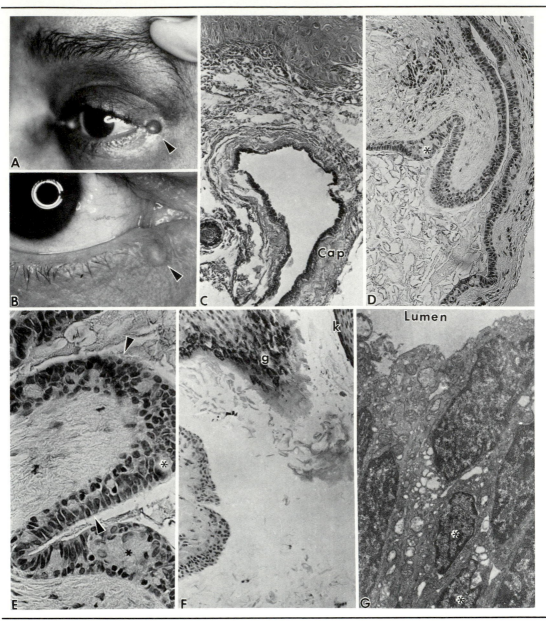

Figure 5.5
Moll's gland cyst. In A and B, dome-shaped, semi-transparent cysts are seen in typical inner or outer canthus locations (arrowheads). In C, a dermal cystic space is surrounded with a layer of compressed collagenous (Cap) tissue. In D and E, the two-layer structure is similar to apocrine hidrocystoma; however, the peripheral cells or basal cells of the cyst wall are not myoepithelial cells. The luminal cells are either secretory cells (arrowheads in E) or keratinizing ductal cells (k in F) with formation of keratohyalin granules (g in F). Large clear cells (* in D and E) are either clustered or sporadically distributed. These cells are PAS positive. The cyst may contain keratinous debris (D–F). In G, electron microscopy of part of the wall revealed secretory-type luminal cells with numerous secretory vacuoles. The second layer cells (*) are not myoepithelial cells. (C, × 48; D, × 60; E and F, × 152; G, × 6,975.) (Courtesy of George A. Youngberg, M.D.)

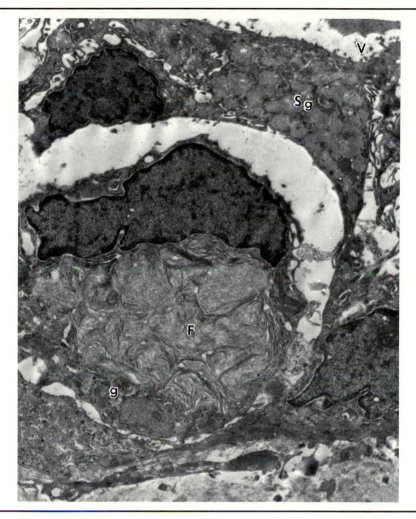

Figure 5.6
Moll's gland cyst. The large clear cell contains a mass of filamentous aggregation (F) and glycogen particles (g). A luminal cell has secretory granules (Sg) and long, sparse villi (V). (× 7,400.) (Courtesy of George A. Youngberg, M.D.)

more duct-like structures may connect to the epidermis, either directly or through a dilated hair follicle. Some lumina are round and dilated while others are thick walled and show papilliferous epithelial structures; so much so that the tumors resemble syringocystadenoma papilliferum. In fact, in some areas the tumor stroma may show an infiltration of lymphocytes and plasma cells similar to those seen in syringocystadenoma papilliferum (Fig. 5.7G). Dilated apocrine glands may be seen between or beneath the tumor masses. In some cases, the covering epidermis shows verrucous hyperplasia compatible with the picture of an organoid nevus.[19,20]

In apocrine adenoma[23,24] tubular structures and lumen formation are less

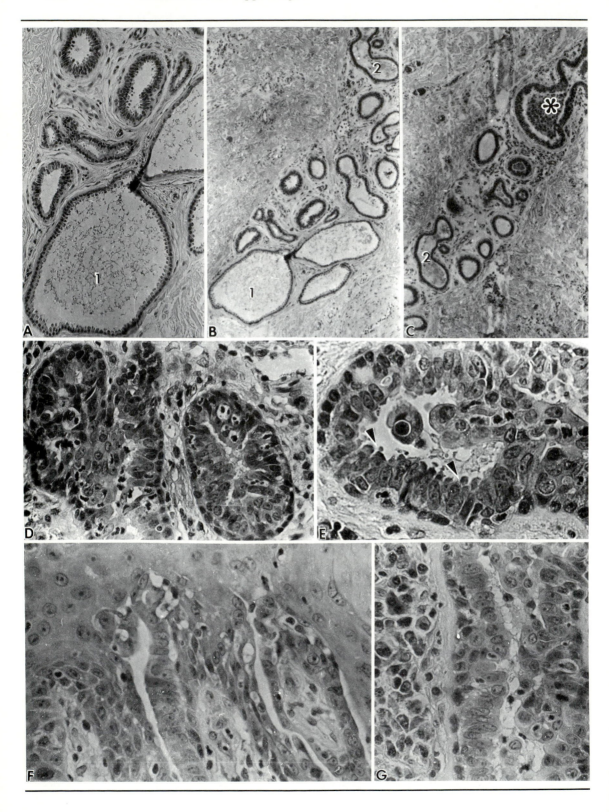

prominent, and tufts of luminal cells form papillary projections and protrude into the large lumina (Fig. 5.7E). Large lumina may be filled with an adenomatous growth and sometimes difficult to differentiate from apocrine adenocarcinoma.[27–29]

In apocrine fibroadenoma the histologic picture is very similar to that of intracanalicular fibroadenoma of the breast.[25,26] Cleft-like spaces lined by two layers of epithelial cells are embedded in abundant fibrous stroma. The basal cells are cuboidal or flat, and the luminal cells are columnar with eosinophilic cytoplasm and apparent decapitation secretion. Cleft-like spaces may be largely occluded by proliferation of wall cells and are occasionally dilated, forming small cystic spaces.

Histochemistry

The eccrine type of enzymes in tubular apocrine adenoma are either negative, weakly positive, or irregularly reactive, whereas the apocrine type (acid phosphatase, indoxyesterase) are strongly positive.[19] Fluorescent lipid granules are abundant in apical cytoplasm of luminal cells.[19]

Electron Microscopy

In tubular apocrine adenoma the luminal cells exhibit decapitation secretion and contain annulate lamellar structures, both of which are characteristic of apocrine secretory cells. However, large, dense apocrine-type secretory granules are undeveloped, and myoepithelial cells are not differentiated.[19]

Apocrine Adenocarcinoma

Carcinomas of apocrine glands occur most frequently in apocrine areas of the body, particularly in the axilla.[24,28–35] In nevus sebaceus not only benign varieties of apocrine adenomas but apocrine adenocarcinoma may also develop secondarily.[21] Some of the extramammary Paget's disease may represent an epidermotropic apocrine adenocarcinoma (see Fig. 5.20A, B, C), discussed on page 174. Apocrine adenocarcinomas are rare tumors: Baes and Suurmond[28] collected 18 cases from the literature including their own. Within their list are

Figure 5.7
Apocrine adenoma and apocrine tubular adenoma. Dilated apocrine glands (cystadenoma) (A) are connected with the proliferative area (B) and the adenomatous (in C) portion. In A, B, and C the numbered structures (1, 2) correspond to each other in the three serial pictures. In D and E, a higher magnification of adenomatous or even epitheliomatous lesions are shown; decapitation secretion (arrowheads in E) is seen. In F and G, more tubular lesions (tubular adenoma) are demonstrated. (A, × 130; B and C, × 65; D–G, × 520.)*

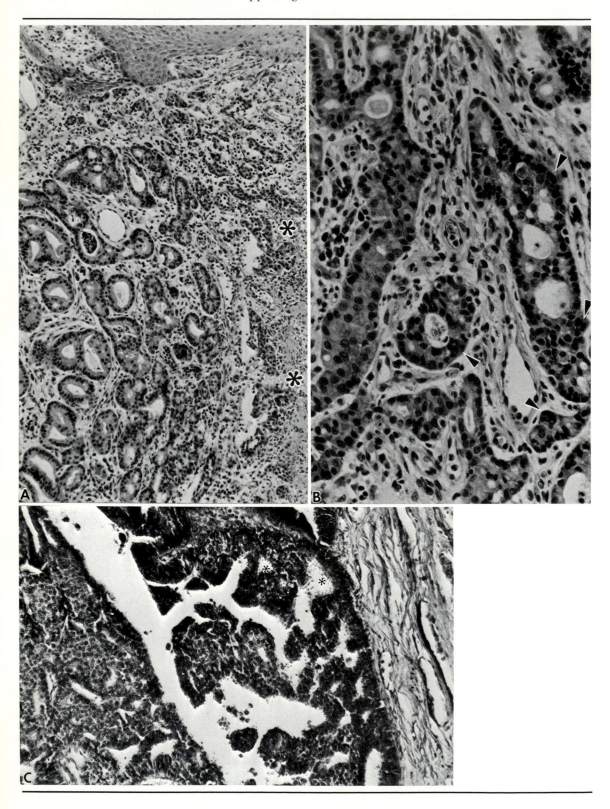

some cases of extramammary Paget's disease. Warkel and Helwig[24] reported 10 cases of axillary apocrine adenocarcinomas. The other cases reported have all been sporadic ones.[29–35] In Warkel and Helwig's series, tumor size ranged from 1.5 to 8.0 cm. They occurred singly or multiply and presented as nodular or cystic masses. The covering skin was red to purple and occasionally ulcerated. Although the tumors often produced discomfort, they did not cause pain. With the exception of one lesion of 30 years' duration, most cases had a history of one year or less. Patients' ages ranged from 25 to 91 years; however, only two patients were younger than 40 years, and the mean age was 57.9 years. The male to female ratio was 5:3, and cases were distributed equally among whites and blacks. The mortality rate of apocrine carcinoma was relatively low, in the range of 39%,[2] and may reflect the difficulty in differentiating, histologically, apocrine adenoma, which is benign, from apocrine adenocarcinoma.

Histology

The excised tumors are red or reddish brown and most are firm and solid, but cystic and hemorrhagic foci are occasionally observed.[23] Microscopic pictures vary from those that are similar to apocrine adenoma to those adenocarcinomas that are poorly differentiated. In most tumors a fairly well differentiated portion, moderately differentiated areas, and foci of poor differentiation can be found (Fig. 5.8). More differentiated areas tend to form complex glandular patterns in which apocrine-like large lumina with single to multilayered luminal cells are present. Cytoplasm is eosinophilic; decapitation secretion is evident at least in some areas[35]; and PAS-positive and diastase-resistant granules[32] and often iron-positive granules[33] like those present in a normal apocrine gland may be seen. In moderately differentiated tumors papillary projections or disorganized gland-like tubular structures are encountered (Fig. 5.8B). In poorly differentiated areas more solid epithelial components are present.

Although it may be difficult to determine apocrine origin or differentiation in these tumors, one may still find some areas, often in the uppermost portion, in which apocrine-like features such as a large lumen and tall luminal cells with an evidence of decapitation secretion are present[2,24] (Fig. 5.8C). In addition to this general pattern of growth, one must pay attention to the nuclear atypia (Fig. 5.8B), hyperchromasia, pleomorphism, and mitotic figures when grading apocrine malignancies. Many of these tumors show stromal fibrosis and hyalinization.

Figure 5.8
Apocrine gland carcinoma. In A, a relatively mature and adenomatous area is seen on the left and a more atypical and invasive area (*) is present on the right. In B, high magnification shows some malignant features such as lack of glandular organization and clustered hyperchromatic nuclei (arrowheads); however, very malignant features such as great cellular atypia and mitotic figures are not evident. In C, a more cellular and disorganized tumor still shows decapitation secretion (*). (A and C, × 130; B, × 200.)

Hidradenoma Papilliferum

This rare tumor is very unique in that generally only women over 30 (average 44)[7] are affected. The majority occur in the labia majora, perineal, or perianal areas. Rarely it may be found on the nipple,[36] the eyelid[37] and in the external auditory canal.[38] Interestingly, even these extragenital tumors occurred in females. However, this tumor is extremely rare in black women. The growth, covered with normal skin, has an average size of 0.5 cm (range from 0.1 to 1.0 cm).[39] Malignant transformation was reported in one case in which a fatal metastasizing squamous cell carcinoma developed in a perianal lesion.[40]

Histology

Hidradenoma papilliferum is a good name for this tumor because it is a large apocrine adenoma with papillary projection and proliferation. A fibrous capsule surrounds the entire periphery of the tumor and extends into the tumor along with papillary projections of the wall. Its basic structure is that of a large cyst in which the wall epithelium has proliferated to produce an adenoma (Fig. 5.9). The wall epithelium near the epidermis may undergo an epidermal type of keratinization (Fig. 5.9) or may consist of a single layer of flattened cells. Although the epidermal connection may not be obvious in most tumors, these features suggest that the upper part of the cyst was once open to the surface. The lower part of the wall protrudes into the cystic space in the form of multiple papillary projections. Within the proliferative papillary structure numerous tubular, glandular, or slit-like lumina are formed and anastomosed to each other; the tubular structures thus produced are lined with eosinophilic, tall columnar cells of apocrine type on the luminal side and cuboidal cells along the basal layer. Most of the latter cells are myoepithelial cells. The luminal cells show decapitation secretion.

Histochemistry

The luminal cells contain a number of large, PAS-positive, diastase-resistant granules. Nonspecific esterase, acid phosphatase, and other apocrine enzymes are positive, whereas eccrine enzymes such as phosphorylase are negative. Myoepithelial cells can be demonstrated with alkaline phosphatase.[36]

Electron Microscopy

In the luminal cells lipid granules, dense secretory granules, and decapitation secretion of the apical portion are demonstrated. Myofilament-rich myoepithelial cells are found along the periphery and correspond to the cuboidal basal cells.[36,41]

Syringocystadenoma Papilliferum

This tumor can occur singly or as part of an organoid nevus (nevus sebaceus) (see p. 131). In either case it is found most frequently on the scalp or on the

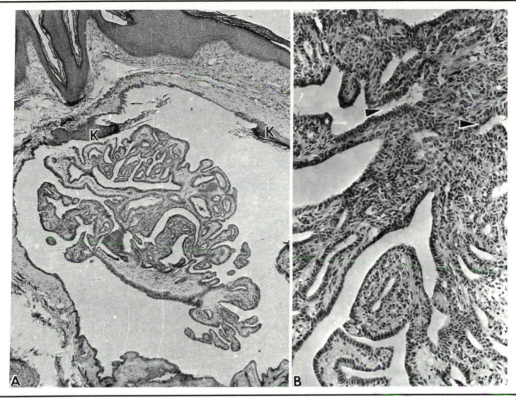

Figure 5.9
Hidradenoma papilliferum. In A, an intradermal cyst contains projections. The cyst wall near the epidermis is keratinized (K), whereas the rest is covered with apocrine-type tall epithelium. In B, a papillary projection is covered with apocrine secretory epithelium (arrowheads). (A, × 65; B, × 163.)

face and in only about one-fourth of the cases does it occur in the other locations.[42] When associated with an organoid nevus, it begins early in life as a moist, keratotic nodule within a linear[43] or zosteriform[44] lesion. At puberty it starts growing faster and produces a verrucous, vegetative, papillomatous lesion that often exudes a secretion and becomes crusted (hidradénome verruqueux fistulo-végétant; wet wart). Those lesions not associated with an organoid nevus may appear during puberty or later in life.

Histology
Usually one to several openings are seen going through an acanthotic and hyperkeratotic epidermis (Fig. 5.10A, D). The openings may lead to a large cystic space extending deep into the dermis. As the name of the tumor indicates, papilliferous projections extend into the main cyst from the cyst wall (Fig. 5.10A). In some tumors such growths occupy most of the cystic space, while in others the cystic spaces are almost empty. In still others cyst formation is not prominent, and only narrow or slightly dilated and branching

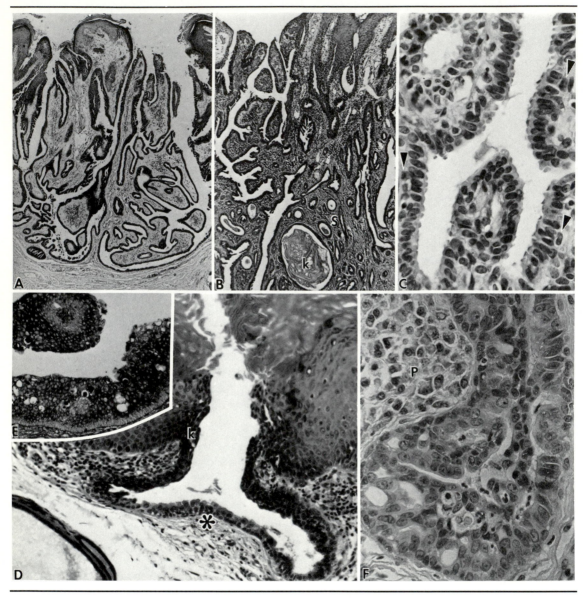

Figure 5.10
Syringocystadenoma papilliferum. In A, large cystic spaces extend from the epidermis down and contain papilliferous projections. In B, syringoma-like spaces (S) and large cysts containing keratin (k) underlie the main lesion. In C, typically apocrine-type epithelium lines the tubular cystic spaces; the luminal cells are tall and columnar, and the basal cells are round or cuboidal (arrowheads). In D, the cyst wall near the opening to the epidermis is covered with keratinized epithelium (k), which gradually changes in deeper portions into columnar epithelium (*). In E, this portion of the wall cells and a papillary projection are strongly PAS (glycogen) positive. In F, a more adenomatous portion is surrounded with a heavy infiltration of plasma cells (P). (A, × 31; B, × 62; C, × 155; D and E, × 95; F, × 494.)

tubular spaces are present (Fig. 5.10B, C). Syringoma-like structures and cysts containing keratin may be part of the lesion (Fig. 5.10B).

The cyst wall close to or continuous with the epidermal invagination is composed of stratified keratinocytes without any feature of glandular cells (Fig. 5.10D). Deeper into the tumor the cyst wall epithelium gradually becomes taller, columnar, and eosinophilic, and thus resembles apocrine secretory cells (Fig. 5.10C, D). The surface of the papilliferous projections and anastomosing tubulocystic spaces formed within the projections are covered with the same secretory cells. The basal cells on which these secretory cells stand are round to cuboidal. The stroma is heavily infiltrated with plasma cells (Fig. 5.10F); in fact, this feature may be used to differentiate the tumor from apocrine cystadenoma, tubular apocrine adenoma, and erosive adenomatosis of nipple, and other lesions. Apocrine glands, either normal or dilated, are often present under the lesion and a connection with the tumor may be demonstrated by step sections. A dilated apocrine gland underlying the tumor may contain papillary or even adenomatous growths and may thus resemble apocrine cystadenoma or even apocrine adenoma on a small scale.

Histochemistry and Electron Microscopy

The luminal cells may contain glycogen (Fig. 5.10E), phosphorylase, and succinic dehydrogenase.[16] In all three lesions so far tested eccrine-specific monoclonal antibodies EKH5 and EKH6 were positive.[14] Gigantic apocrine-type secretory granules and annulate lamellae are absent. Dense secretory granules are more like those found in the mucous cells of the eccrine gland. Intracytoplasmic cavity formation, commonly observed in the embryonic stage of acrosyringeal duct formation and in several tumors differentiating toward eccrine structures, is frequently observed (Fig. 5.11C). Some part of the cyst wall undergoes keratinization (Fig. 5.11D) as seen in an acrosyringeal eccrine duct or in syringoma (see Fig. 2.25C). Although high columnar cells show a basally located large nucleus, Golgi apparatus and, among other apocrine features, decapitation secretion (Fig. 5.11A, B), this tumor does not show definite apocrine differentiation. Cuboidal basal cells are also typical myoepithelial cell-like because of their general configuration and the deep invagination of their nuclear membrane (Fig. 5.11A) but they do not contain visible myofilaments; these basal cells may be immature myoepithelial cells.

It is indeed possible that this is an apocrine tumor but such an immature one that neither secretory granules nor myoepithelial cells have been fully developed. Alternatively, this may be an eccrine tumor that shows some apocrine features such as decapitation secretion. In sweat gland tumors decapitation-like mode of secretion is also seen in eccrine tumors such as eccrine spiradenoma (Fig. 2.39). A third position worth considering is that in an immature neoplasm, such as syringocystadenoma papilliferum, dermal cylindroma, or even basal cell epithelioma, the degree of differentiation is so minimal that the pluripotential matrix cells may differentiate in two or more directions. The recent discovery of "apoeccrine gland" and its impact on appendage tumors of sweat gland origin or differentiation will be discussed on p. 183.

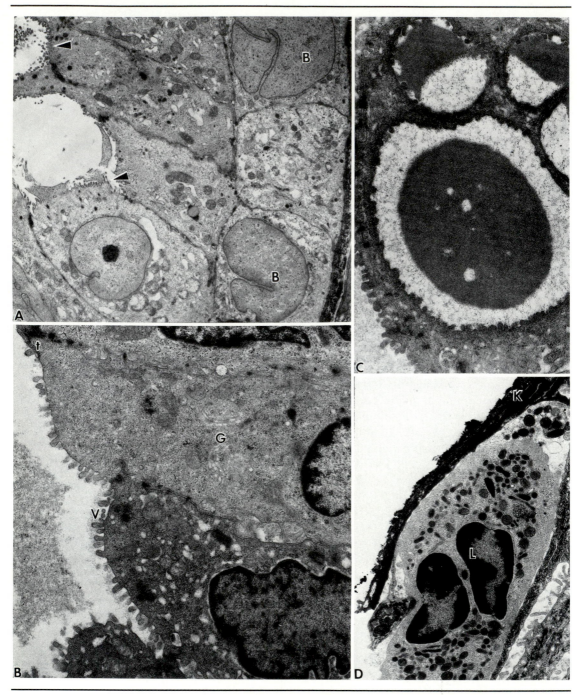

Figure 5.11

Syringocystadenoma papilliferum. In A, round basal cells (B) with a notched nuclear membrane and luminal cells showing decapitation secretion of apical cytoplasm by forming chained vesicles (arrowheads) are observed. The secretory cells that show decapitation do not contain large secretory granules. In B, secretory cells are magnified to show the luminal villi (V), luminal tight junctions (t), Golgi apparatus (G), and numerous vesicles. In C, intracytoplasmic cavity formation is seen. In D, keratinized luminal cells (K) are lifted up by a migratory leukocyte (L). (A, × 1,900; B and C, × 9,025; D, × 3,088.)

Dermal Cylindroma

The classic dermal cylindroma occurs as multiple nodular lesions on the scalp and is dominantly inherited. The lesions first appear early in life and increase in number and size with advancing age. It eventually covers the scalp with nodules and tumors of various sizes as a turban is wrapped around the head; hence, the name "turban tumor" (Fig. 5.12). These tumors are smooth surfaced, flesh colored, and often become the size of a golf ball or larger. Occasionally the lesions are found on the face, in the external ear canal, and even on the trunk and extremities.[45,46] Hairs entangled between tumors and their secretion make it difficult to clean the scalp, and promote bacterial growth such that some patients seek medical treatment because of the intolerable fetid odor caused by the secondary infection.

Solitary lesions on the scalp or on the face that begin in adulthood have been reported to be as common as multiple lesions[47]; however, it is sometimes difficult to clearly differentiate this tumor from an eccrine spiradenoma. Also reported is coexistence with eccrine spiradenoma in the same lesion.[47,48] Single, tender lesions in a patient without a family history of this tumor[48] could represent a dermal cylindroma-like variation of eccrine spiradenoma. More logical, however, is the association of multiple cylindroma and multiple

Figure 5.12
Dermal cylindroma. The scalp is covered with papulonodular lesions and tumors; the lesions are distributed like a turban. The patient has a few lesions on the nasolabial folds, a typical location for trichoepitheliomas (see Fig. 3.17A, B).

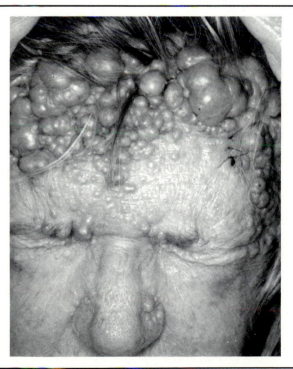

trichoepithelioma[47,49–55] since both are autosomal dominant diseases, and if one considers dermal cylindroma an apocrine tumor, both are derived from the hair germs in fetal development. In these cases the scalp lesions are typical dermal cylindroma, whereas the facial lesions are an admixture of both.

Histology

Numerous epithelial islands of various sizes are clustered in the dermis and extend into the subcutis (Fig. 5.13A). No special capsule surrounds the whole tumor but individual islands are surrounded with a thick hyalin membrane (Fig. 5.13B). In a three-dimensional picture obtained by serial sections and reconstruction of images, it can be seen that each group of tumor islands are mostly continuous as are the hyalin membranes. When the hyalin membrane proliferates much more than does the epithelial growth of the tumor, it in- vaginates into the tumor parenchyma (Fig. 5.13E) and in some areas becomes entangled with the tumor cells. When small invaginations are cross-sectioned, they are demonstrated to be hyalin droplets. Hyalin membranes and droplets can be delineated clearly with PAS stain (Fig. 5.14A, B). The well-fitting ar- rangement of various-sized and shaped tumor islands separated by the septate of hyalin membranes looks like a jigsaw puzzle.[56] The tumor islands have two types of cells: along the hyalin membrane small basaloid cells, often palisad- ing, and larger but less basophilic (pale) cells, present toward the center (Fig. 5.13E, F). In some tumors lumen formation within the islands is frequent (Fig. 5.13), while in others it is very difficult to find luminal differentiation. Some lumina are very similar—tall and columnar and showing decapitation secre- tion—to the apocrine secretory segment while others resemble the eccrine secretory segment.

Histochemistry

The eccrine type of enzymes are found negative in this tumor. A weak reaction of apocrine enzymes such as acid phosphatase and β-glucuronidase may sug- gest apocrine differentiation.[57,58] As in syringocystadenoma papilliferum, poor differentiation of tumor cells makes it difficult to classify this tumor as either an apocrine or eccrine neoplasm. As discussed previously (p. 57), decapita- tion secretion is not an absolute criterion for apocrine differentiation. Nerve

Figure 5.13
Dermal cylindroma. In A, epithelial islands of various shapes and sizes are present in the dermis. Some islands have cystic spaces (C). In B, a thick hyalin membrane (H) surrounds most islands. One island has a ductal lumen (*). In C, another ductal space is found (*). In D, eccrine glands (e) are incorporated into the stroma. In E, palisading peripheral cells and invagination of hyalin membranes (arrowheads) into the parenchyma are observed. Some tumor cells show clear cytoplasm (c). In F, some luminal cells of the cystic space show decapitation secretion (*), whereas slit-like spaces apparently continuous to this lumen resemble an eccrine gland (e). Hyalin droplets (h) and palisading basaloid cells (B) can also be noticed at the periphery. (A, × 33; B, C, E, and F, × 613; D, × 130.)

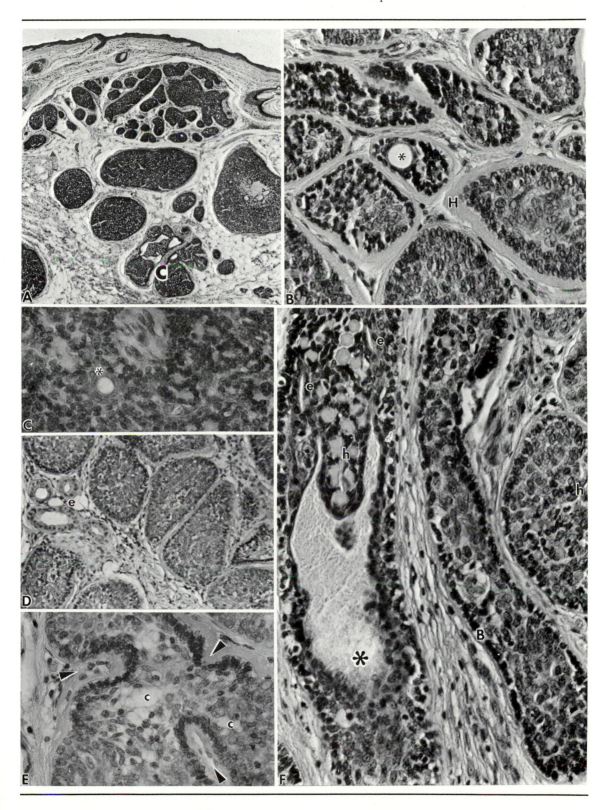

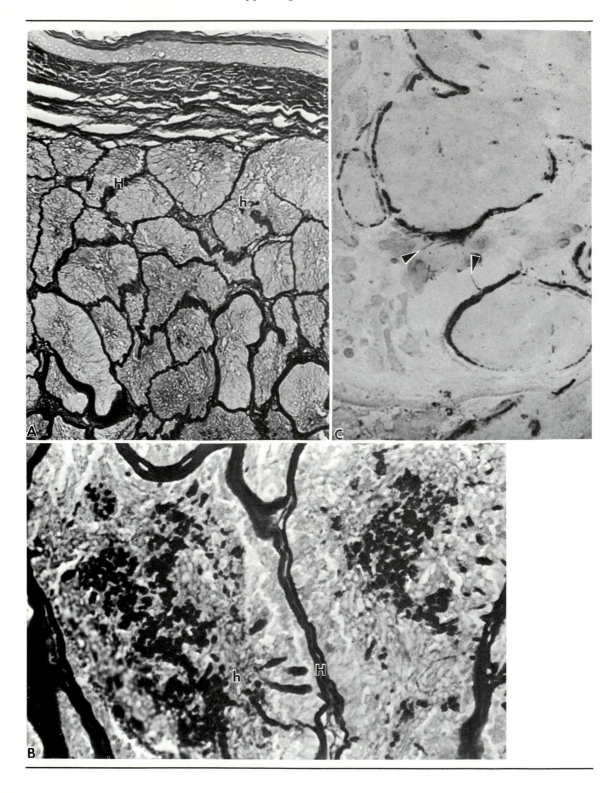

bundles demonstrated with acetylcholinesterase stain tightly surround most tumor islands (Fig. 5.14C).

Electron Microscopy

Most of the centrally located, pale, large cells do not show definite cellular markers, either for ductal or glandular epithelium. In other words, these are indeterminate cells (Fig. 5.15). Some cells are arranged around lumina where the luminal villi are either ductal or secretory (Fig. 5.16). The secretory granules if present, could be of the eccrine mucous (dark) cell type[59,60] or of two types, one being large and containing lipid globules and the other being mitochondrial, resembling apocrine secretory cells (Fig. 5.16 and Table 1.4). Decapitation secretion has also been confirmed.[61] A large number of Langerhans cells migrate between tumor cells (Fig. 5.15). The hyalin membrane is composed of a large portion of loosely organized amorphous material identical to basal lamina substance and an admixture of fine collagen and anchoring fibrils (Fig. 5.17). The presence of anchoring fibrils is interesting because they are practically absent in the basal lamina that surrounds the eccrine, apocrine, and hair follicle structures.

Malignant Cylindroma

Malignant transformation of dermal cylindroma is rare but 10 cases have been reported.[62–71] Multiple[62–69] as well as solitary tumors[68,69,71] have metastasized to superficial lymph nodes[65,68] and/or to viscera.[62–64,66,67,69,70] Intracranial invasion has been reported in three cases.[66,67,71]

Histology

In the malignant area of the tumor the peripheral palisading pattern, dual cell population, and loss of hyalin membrane are frequently cited. The small basophilic cells along the periphery are replaced with large pale cells that often contain prominent nucleoli. Mitotic figures vary from scanty to numerous. Cellular atypia, hyperchromatism of the nucleus, atypical mitosis, and other signs of malignancy may be minimal. In many instances an island-forming pattern is still maintained although the thick hyalin membrane is reduced to a thin band of basement membrane.

Figure 5.14
Dermal cylindroma. In A and B, PAS stain with diastase digestion demonstrates neutral mucopolysaccharides in the hyalin membranes (H) that surround the whole tumor as well as individual tumor islands. Hyalin droplets (h) are also stained. In C, acetylcholinesterase stain demonstrates a thick ring of nerve bundles surrounding most of the large tumor islands. Small fibers (arrowheads) are also stained. (A, × 65; B, × 400; C, × 33.)

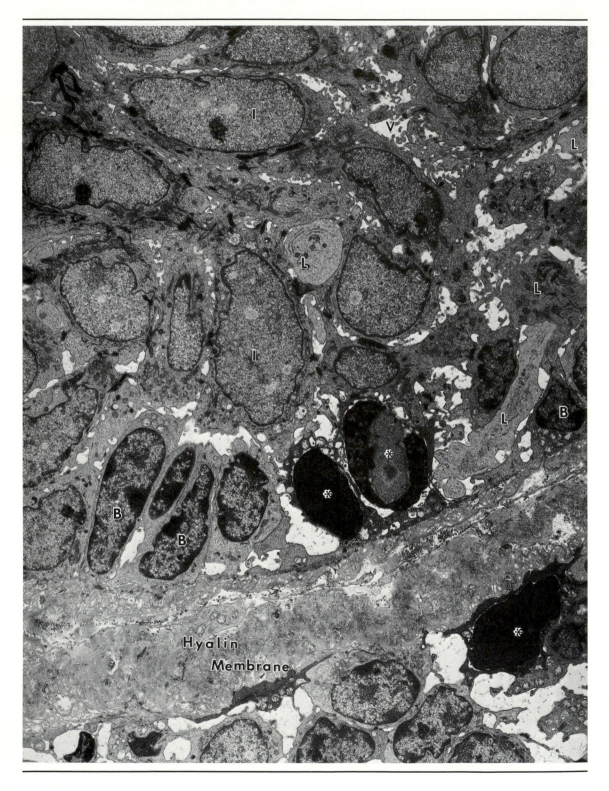

Figure 5.15
Dermal cylindroma. Small peripheral cells or basaloid cells (B) as seen on light microscopy have dense nuclear chromatin and are often pyknotic (*). The centrally located indeterminate cells (I) correspond to large pale cells of light microscopy; they may differentiate some villi (V) but not lumen in this picture. Langerhans cells are abundant (L). The thick hyalin membrane separates this tumor island from the one below it. At this magnification only predominantly amorphous substances are resolved within the hyalin membrane. (× 4,250.)

Figure 5.16
Dermal cylindroma. Luminal cells differentiate villi (V) and apocrine-type secretory granules composed of vacuoles (v) and a dense substance (*). Other granules are electron light and are derived from mitochondrion (m). n—nucleus. (× 25,000.)

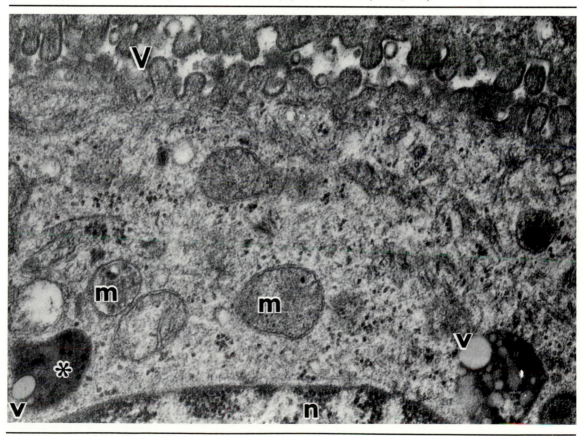

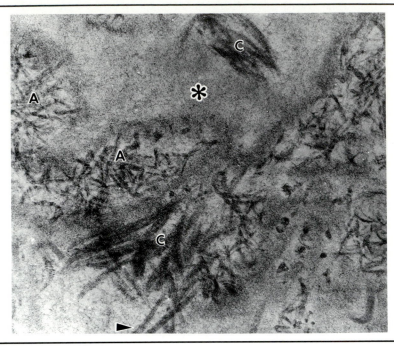

Figure 5.17
Dermal cylindroma. The hyalin membrane is composed mainly of an amorphous substance (*) identical to that of basal lamina. Enmeshed in it one finds aggregated anchoring fibrils (A), split collagen (C) and thin collagen fibers (arrowhead). (× 36,000.)

Erosive Adenomatosis of the Nipple or Florid Papillomatosis of the Nipple Ducts

This is an adenomatous growth of the major nipple ducts with a clinical picture very similar to that of Paget's disease. An erosive, crusted, eczematous lesion on the nipple may show a blood-stained or serous discharge.[72–74] Nodular enlargement of the nipple develops at a later stage.

Histology
Several invaginations of acanthotic epidermis lead into tubulocystic spaces in the dermis (Fig. 5.18). The overall picture is thus similar to syringocystadenoma papilliferum or tubular apocrine adenoma.[72] Considering the mammary gland as a modified apocrine gland, this tumor may represent the lactiferous duct counterpart of these apocrine tumors. The tubular ducts are lined with a luminal layer of tall columnar cells and a peripheral layer of small, dense cuboidal cells (Fig. 5.18C). Decapitation secretion and secretory products in the lumen are also observed[73,75] (Fig. 5.18C). As in syringocystadenoma papilliferum, the squamous cell epithelium may cover the luminal surface near the invagination of the epidermis[73,74] (Fig. 5.18A). No cytologic signs of ma-

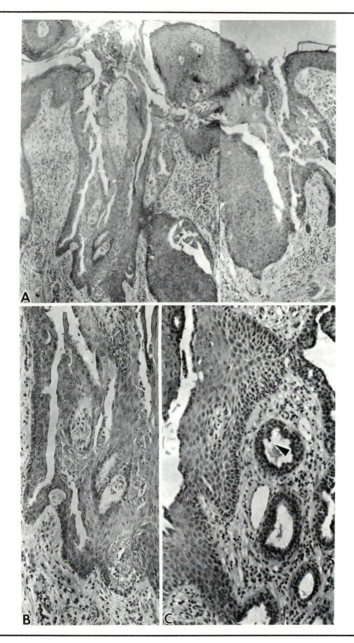

Figure 5.18
*Erosive adenomatosis of the nipple. In A, invagination of the epidermis is trans-
formed into tubulocystic structures similar to those seen in syringocystadenoma papilliferum (Fig. 5.10). In B and C, the wall epithelium near the opening is a stratified
squamous type, whereas deeper parts and a tubulocystic lesion are walled with an
apocrine-type tall cell; in such areas decapitation secretion (arrowhead in C) and cellular debris in the lumina are observed. (A, × 65; B, × 130; C, × 163.)*

lignancy are present and in this regard this tumor can be differentiated from the intraductal carcinoma of the breast.[74]

Paget's Disease

Paget's disease begins on the nipple or areola as a unilateral, sharply defined erythematous and eczematous plaque with surface exudation and crusting. The lesion eventually spreads to the surrounding skin areas beyond the areola. An intraductal or invasive carcinoma of the underlying breast is almost always present. It is, however, still controversial as to which condition is the primary disease, the breast duct carcinoma or the intraepidermal Paget's cells. When a palpable mass is felt in the breast, axillary lymph node metastasis is found in about two-thirds of the patients.[76] Lymph node metastasis may[76] or may not[77] be found without an underlying palpable mass. Male patients have been reported[78]; one patient developed Paget's disease after estrogen therapy for a prostatic cancer.[79]

Extramammary Paget's Disease

Skin lesions clinically and histologically identical to mammary Paget's disease can occur in the anogenital region and axilla. The histologic pagetoid phenomenon within the surface epithelium is also observed in the external ear canal[80] in association with ceruminous gland carcinoma and in the eyelid with Moll's gland carcinoma.[81] The most common site of extramammary Paget's disease is the vulva followed by male genitalia.[82] As a very rare association the patient with mammary Paget's disease may also develop a vulvar lesion.[83] Perianal or vulvar lesions can also be secondary to an adenocarcinoma of the rectum or cervix.[84,85] The clinical picture of extramammary Paget's disease is identical to that of mammary Paget's disease but it is often intensely pruritic; it is not uncommon that many patients with this disease are misdiagnosed as having chronic eczema, tinea cruris, and Bowen's disease among others. The recurrence rate of extramammary Paget's disease is high; this may be related to multifocal occurrence of this disease and the presence of an underlying adenocarcinoma.[86]

Histology

The histologic pictures between the mammary and extramammary types are similar. Clear cells with large pale nucleus, that is, Paget's cells, are scattered through the lower layer of the epidermis in "buckshot" distribution (Fig. 5.19). In more advanced lesions the increased Paget's cells in cluster compress the keratinocytes to make them degenerate, so much so that the thin septae of tonofibrils are all that remains of the keratinocytes (Fig. 5.20D). The compressed basal cells are also reduced to a thin layer of tonofibrils and barely holding large group of tumor cells (Fig. 5.20D). In more advanced lesions, the breakage of the barrier of tonofibrillar bands and a spilling-out of Paget's

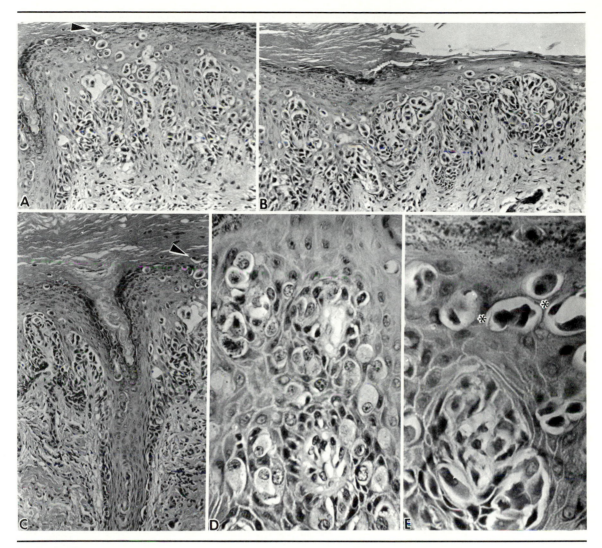

Figure 5.19
Paget's disease. In A and B, large tumor cells give the epidermis a "buckshot" pattern. Some cells are being eliminated (arrowheads in A and C) through the stratum corneum. In C, tumor cells are spreading along the eccrine duct. In D and E, large, pale cells produce retraction spaces between the surrounding keratinocytes and thus appear as if they were floating in empty spaces. Keratinocytes compressed between the tumor cells are reduced into a thin band of tonofibrils (*). (A–C, × 130; D, × 163; E, × 530.)

cells into the dermis are observed. Although the dermal invasion of Paget's cells can occur under the pressure of an increased cell population, the major route of dermal involvement is usually through the seeding of the ductal epithelium of mammary, eccrine, (Fig. 5.19C) and, less frequently, the apocrine ducts and external root sheath of hair follicles. Tumor cells often plug these

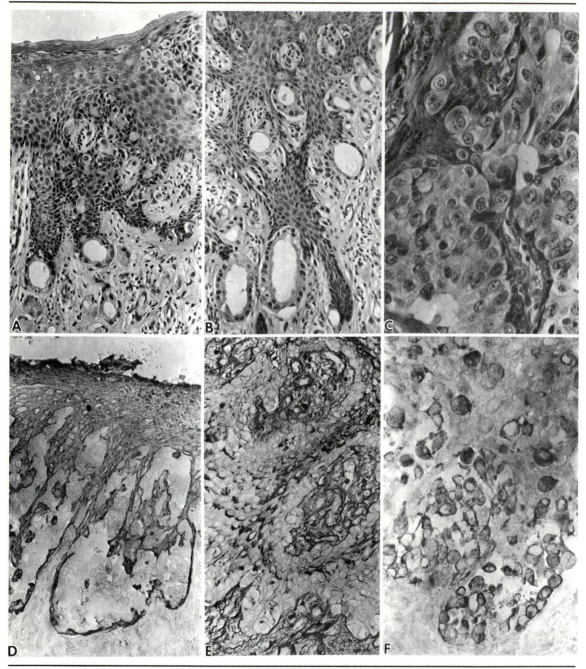

Figure 5.20
Paget's disease. In A, B, and C glandular acini formation is seen in addition to scattered tumor cells. In D, keratin bands holding tumor masses along the dermoepidermal junction and separating tumor masses are stained with EKH4, which recognizes 50 Kd keratin. In E, PAS stain was negative in Paget's cells but glycogen was present within the surrounding epidermal cells. In F, EKH6 is positive in Paget cells. (A, B, and D, × 130; C and F, × 530; E, × 200.)

ducts but do not invade the extraductal tissues; these tumor-plugged ducts are called "comedo carcinoma" (Fig. 5.21). The ductal and follicular epithelium are eventually ruptured and dermal and lymphatic spread follows.

Extramammary Paget's disease shows essentially the same picture as does the mammary type. Most cases of extramammary Paget's disease are not associated with underlying malignancy; in two large series 21 to 24% of the cases showed deeper invasive carcinomas.[87,88] The underlying adenocarcinoma could be of eccrine, apocrine, Bartholin's, periurethral, or perianal gland origin.[89] It is more often observed in this type than in the mammary gland variety that several cells form rosette or glandular acini within the involved epidermis (Fig. 5.20A, B, C). The association of extramammary Paget's disease with a concurrent or nonconcurrent internal malignancy has been established in 29% of cases.[88]

Figure 5.21
Paget's disease. A mammary duct is plugged with tumor cells and debris; this is the picture of "comedo carcinoma." (× 150.) (Courtesy of Martin C. Mihm, Jr., M.D.)

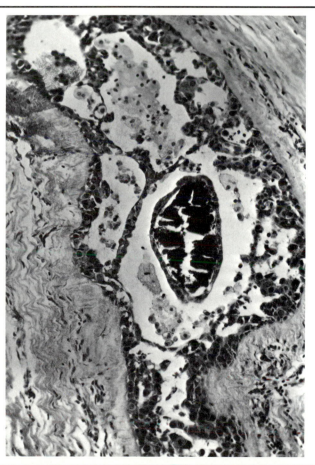

Histochemistry

Neutral mucopolysaccharides demonstrated with PAS stain with diastase digestion has been used to identify some Paget's cells. This stain is negative in the majority of mammary Paget's cells (Fig. 5.20E) and variably positive in the extramammary type; it seems to depend upon whether the lesion is secondary to underlying glandular carcinomas that produce neutral mucopolysaccharides. Acid mucopolysaccharides, mainly sialomucin, are demonstrated with alcian blue (pH 3.0 and 4.5) and digested with sialidase[90] or neuramidase.[91] These stains may detect additional Paget's cells that the H&E stain missed, particularly in the underlying adnexa.

The histogenesis of Paget's disease has been debated for over 100 years without conclusions; more recently, however, immunohistochemical studies have begun to shed some light on this problem. That Paget's cells originate from keratinocytes has been ruled out as it is now known that the carcinoembryonic antigen, which is absent in keratinocytes and present in eccrine and apocrine glands, has been demonstrated in both mammary and genital lesions.[89] In mammary[92] and extramammary[92–94] Paget's disease, cytokeratin species analysis revealed that Paget's cells contain the glandular type of keratin that is seen in apocrine and eccrine secretory epithelia and lack the epidermal and ductal type of keratin. The EKH4 antikeratin monoclonal antibody was positive in the keratinocytes found in the lesions, including the compressed bands of tonofibrils that enmesh Paget's cells, but negative in Paget's cells per se[94] (Fig. 5.20D). The absence of S100 protein, which is always present in melanocytic cells, indicates that no relationship exists between the extramammary Paget's cells and the melanocytes.[95]

The problem of apocrine versus eccrine origin or differentiation is more complex because the results are often contradictory and there are no extensive and coordinated studies comparing mammary and extramammary Paget's disease. Supporting the apocrine nature of extramammary Paget's disease is that gross cystic disease fluid protein (GCDFP-15), which is only present in the secretory and ductal cells of apocrine glands in normal human skin, was demonstrated in 6 out of 7 cases of vulvar, anogenital, and axillary Paget's disease.[2,96,97] The only negative case was one of perianal Paget's disease.[97] GCDFP-15 is a glycoprotein of 15 kd found in the fluid of gross cystic disease of the breast.[98] Except that Paget's disease preferentially affects the so-called apocrine areas of the body, including the mammary gland, and that GCDFP-15 is present in the tumor cells, modern histochemical and immunohistochemical evidence supporting the apocrine theory is rather scanty.

The eccrine differentiation of extramammary Paget's cells has been supported by several lines of histochemical and immunohistochemical evidence. Belcher[99] demonstrated the presence of the eccrine type of enzymes such as amylophosphorylase and succinic dehydrogenase. The reaction pattern of several lectins in genital Paget's cells was similar to that of the eccrine secretory segment in that both had a cell surface layer of *N*-acetyl-D-galactosamine that reacts with DBA (*Dolichos biflorus* agglutinin).[100,101] The EKH5 and EKH6 monoclonal antikeratin antibodies that react with the eccrine gland[16] were positive in scrotal and vulvar Paget's cells[94] (Fig. 5.20F).

Electron Microscopy

There are several types of cells. One shows secretory cell characteristics such as mucous-type multiple light granules and vacuoles, lumen formation, formation of luminal microvilli (Fig. 5.22), and development of intercellular canaliculi (Fig. 5.23) and intracellular cavity formation.[99,102,103–106] The former feature is often seen in the eccrine gland and the latter in fetal development of intraepidermal eccrine duct and eccrine tumors. Some tumor cells contain numerous vacuoles[103] but do not form acinus.[107,108] Those tumor cells that are rich in smooth endoplasmic reticulum but poor in secretory granules are considered to be an immature stage of the latter. In perianal Paget's disease relatively light cells and dark cells exist; the light cells contain a better developed endoplasmic reticulum and Golgi apparatus, whereas the dark cells have more free ribosomes, making these cells electron dense.[108] Intercellular canaliculi are more frequently seen in the dark cells[108] and are absent in the normal apocrine gland. Very large, complex secretory granules such as those seen in mature apocrine secretory cells have not been reported. The presence of tonofilaments and desmosomes does not particularly favor the epidermal keratinocyte origin of the tumor cells because both the duct and secretory portions of eccrine and apocrine glands are composed of modified keratinocytes and, though poorly developed, contain these organelles. It is best to consider Paget's disease to be an intraepidermal adenocarcinoma caused by the proliferation of an epidermotropic carcinoma of either eccrine or apocrine or other glandular origin.

Figure 5.22
Paget's disease. Secretory-type luminal cells bear long, slender villi (V) and contain numerous cytoplasmic vesicles but no secretory granules. (× 15,000.)

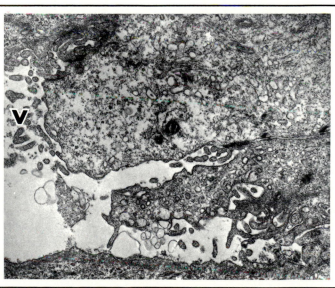

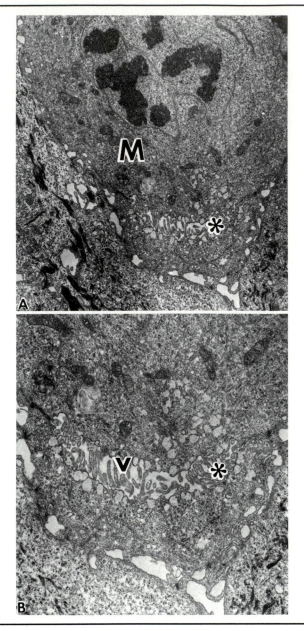

Figure 5.23
Paget's disease. In A, an intercellular canaliculus (*) is produced between a mitotic tumor cell (M) and the neighboring cell. When enlarged (B), long, slender villi (v) cover the luminal surface as in secretory cells. (A, × 6,000; B, × 10,500.)

Apocrine Epithelioma

Apocrine epithelioma, or basal cell epithelioma with apocrine differentiation, has recently been reported by Sakamoto et al.[109] in a 71-year-old Japanese woman. The lesion, 2 by 1.5 cm in diameter, was located in a retroauricular fold behind the earlobe, had gradually grown over 2 years, and more recently had become painful. The surface was irregularly folded and depressed in the center. The invasive tumor involved both the parotid gland and mastoid bone.

Histology

Basaloid cell nests of various sizes and shapes are similar in appearance to basal cell epithelioma. Solid, sclerosing, and adenocystic basal cell epithelioma-like areas are admixed (Fig. 5.24). The stroma is also varied from one area to another; it can be fibrous, sclerosing, or mucinous. The features that separate this tumor from ordinary basal cell epitheliomas are (1) glandular lumen formation: the luminal border is covered with relatively long, slender villi (Fig. 5.25), and some tumor cells containing apocrine-type secretory granules (Table 1.4); (2) the finding of immature myoepithelial cells containing both tonofilaments and myofilaments at the periphery of the tumor island;

Figure 5.24
Apocrine epithelioma. Lumen formation is evident (L) within the basalioma-like epithelial mass. The luminal wall is composed of tall cylindrical cells with basally located nuclei and clear apical cytoplasm. (× 170.) (Courtesy of Fumiko Sakamoto, M.D.)

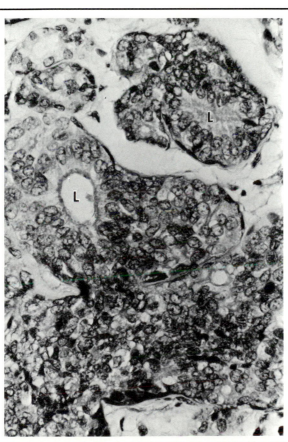

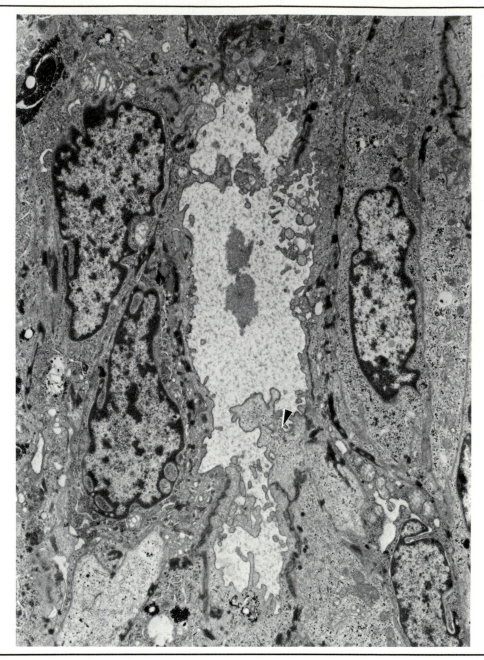

Figure 5.25

Apocrine epithelioma. Although not typically apocrine, these luminal cells show a suggestion of apical cytoplasm decapitation distal to a chain of vesicles (arrowhead) that are forming a demarcation membrane. (× 8,500.) (Courtesy of Fumiko Saka-moto, M.D.)

(3) the presence of apocrine enzymes and the absence of eccrine enzymes (Table 1.3); and (4) the presence of micro-decapitation secretion (Fig. 5.25).

Apoeccrine Gland

A new sweat gland that exhibits a hybrid morphology between apocrine gland and eccrine gland was described by Sato et al. in the human adult

Figure 5.26

In A, apoeccrine gland consists of the secretory coil at the bottom (S); ampulla-like collecting duct (A) in which dense secretory products are retained; dermal duct (D) which is less coiled and relatively straight; and intraepidermal duct (IE). In B, the dermal duct (D) and ampulla portion (A) are enlarged. In C, cross-sections of the secretory coil show an admixture of apocrine-like (Ap) and eccrine-type epithelium (Ec). The former has gigantic secretory granules (*) in tall columnar cells, while the latter has granule-free clear cells (c) and occasional small granules containing dark cells (arrowheads) along the lumen. (A, × 22; B, × 52; C, × 520.)

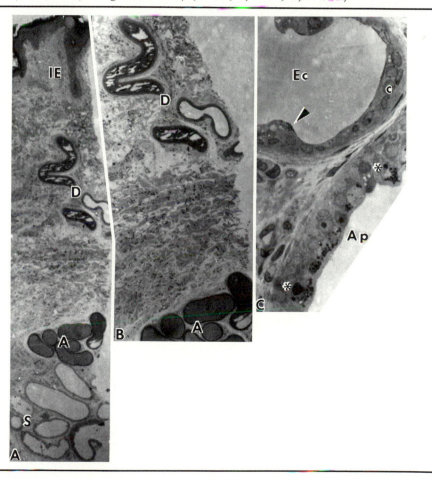

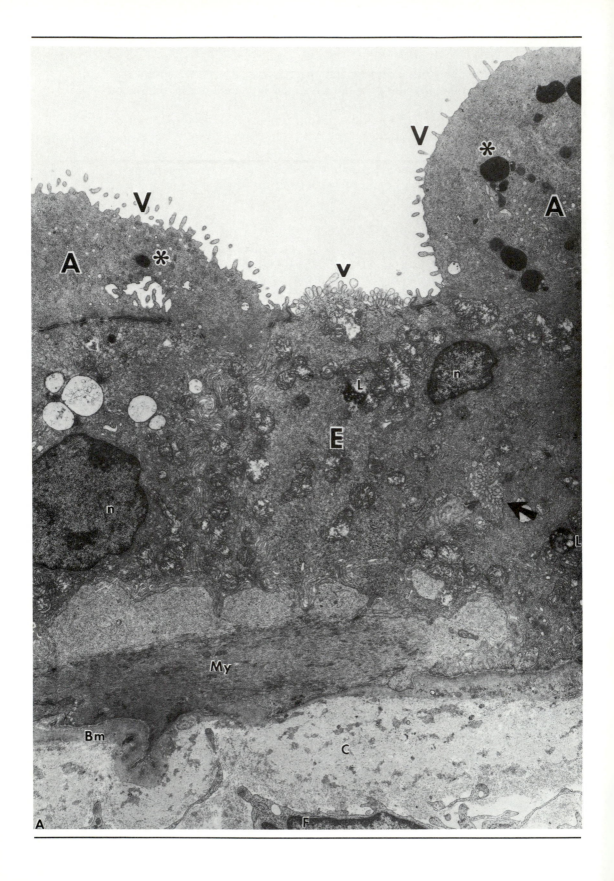

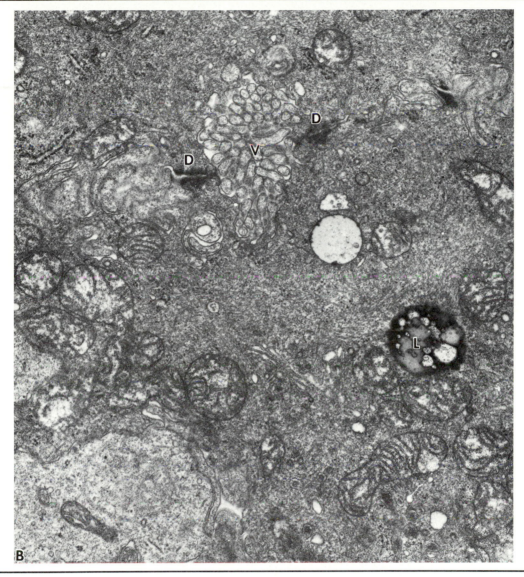

Figure 5.27
In A, apocrine-like cells (A) have large dense granules (∗), round apical swelling and/ or long but sparse luminal villi (V). Eccrine clear cells (E) have no dense granules except lipid granules (L). Clear cells can be identified not only by the absence of dense granules but also the presence of numerous short villi (v) on the luminal surface and intercellular canaliculus (arrow) between two adjoining clear cells. In B, intercellular canaliculus (∗) and lipid granules (L) are enlarged. The former is almost completely filled with villi (V). The canalicular lumen is sealed off from the intercellular spaces by desmosome-tight junction complex (D). Bm—basement membrane; C—collagen; F—fibroblast; My—myoepithelial cell; n—nucleus. (A, × 6,650; B, × 21,000.)

axilla.[110,111] Pharmacological response is eccrine-like and the secretion product is clear and therefore eccrine-like. Sato et al. found that the number of apoeccrine glands increases during puberty in proportion to the decrease of eccrine glands; thus they postulated that the apoeccrine glands develop from the pre-existing eccrine glands.

The importance of the apoeccrine gland in the study of skin appendage tumors is twofold: (1) There are many tumors that exhibit morphologies and (immuno-)histochemical features of both eccrine and apocrine glands. (2) The development of the apoeccrine gland from the eccrine gland suggests that under appropriate conditions such as created in tumorigenesis, tumors that are originally eccrine may be partially or totally differentiated into apocrine tumors and vice versa. In the preceding chapters some difficulties regarding classifying sweat gland tumors were mentioned because they exhibit hybrid features between eccrine and apocrine glands at light microscopic, electron microscopic, and (immuno-)histochemical levels. Examples are apocrine hydrocystoma or cystadenoma (p. 147), tubular apocrine adenoma (p. 153), syringocystadenoma papilliferum (p. 163), and extramammary Paget's disease (p. 178).

Histology

The general architecture of the apoeccrine gland is similar to the apocrine gland except that its duct connects to the epidermis (Fig. 5.26A) instead of hair follicles and a large ampulla forms between the secretory tubule and the straight dermal duct (Fig. 5.26B). The secretory tubule is situated at the junction between the lower dermis and the subcutaneous fat tissue and coiled upon itself many folds (Fig. 5.26A). Two types of lumen are revealed in the cross-section: (1) dilated lumina surrounded by tall wall cells which have large, dense secretory granules (Fig. 5.26C) and often show decapitation secretion. These glands are therefore apocrine in their morphology. (2) small lumina in which the wall epithelium is relatively low and clear without large dense granules (Fig. 5.26C). These are identical to eccrine glands. The entire secretory coil, which is embedded in a dense connective tissue stroma, is connected to an ampulla-like segment which is coiled several times (Fig. 5.26A, B). In this portion of the tubule the luminal surface is lined with a dense ring of filament bundle forming a cuticle-like band. The ampulla may retain secretion products (Fig. 5.26B). The ampulla connects to the straight dermal duct which leads to the epidermal ridge and then to the intraepidermal duct (Fig. 5.26A, B).

Immunohistochemistry

Enzyme histochemistry of this gland has not been studied. Immunohistochemical staining using EKH5 and EKH6 (Table 1.5) revealed that the small eccrine-like portion is always positively stained. In the apocrine-like segment, however, there are variable patterns of staining: in some of these large dilated glands, small segments of the wall are reactive with EKH5 and EKH6. However, sometimes the entire wall epithelium is positively stained. The reactivity with EKH5 and EKH6 suggests that the apoeccrine gland retains eccrine characteristics despite its drastic changes of morphology during adolescence. It would not be surprising if future studies reveal that enzyme histochemical patterns follow the same mixed reaction pattern of eccrine and apocrine differentiation.

Ultrastructure

There are eccrine-like as well as apocrine-like portions. In addition, an admixture of eccrine clear (serous) cells and apocrine secretory cells is observed in some segments (Fig. 5.27A). The proof that those clear cells are similar to or identical to the clear cells of the normal eccrine gland comes from two observations: (1) these cells are rich in glycogen and often contain dense lipid granules (Fig. 5.27A) and (2) there are intercellular canaliculi (Fig. 5.27B). No cells correspond ultrastructurally to dark (mucous) cells of normal eccrine gland in such portion of apocrine and eccrine mixture. It is assumed that the dark cells of the eccrine gland become apocrine-like cells in which mucous granules became large apocrine secretory granules and the decapitation secretion became the mode of their secretion. If this assumption is correct, the decapitation secretion described in putative eccrine tumors such as eccrine spiradenoma and syringocystadenoma papilliferum may be explained. Furthermore, in neoplastic transformation the eccrine dark (mucous) cells may develop into apocrine-like tumor cells. Thus, ultrastructural criteria to distinguish between eccrine and apocrine tumors could become obscure or meaningless. It is, therefore, important to evaluate the neoplasm from an overall picture and not based on one or two specific features such as decapitation secretion.

REFERENCES

1. Mazoujian G, Pinkus GS, David S, Haagensen DE Jr. Immunohistochemistry of a gross cystic disease fluid protein (GCDFP-15) of the breast: A marker of apocrine epithelium and breast carcinomas with apocrine features. Am J Pathol 1983;110:105–112.

2. Warkel RL. Selected apocrine neoplasms. J Cutan Pathol 1984;11:437–449.

3. Morioka S. The natural history of nevus sebaceus. J Cutan Pathol 1985;12:200–213.

4. Civatte J, Tsoitis G, Preaux J. Le naevus apocrine. Ann Dermatol Syph 1974;101:251–261.

5. Rabens SF, Naness JI, Gottlieb BF. Apocrine gland organic hamartoma (apocrine nevus). Arch Dermatol 1976;112:520–522.

6. Vakilzadeh F, Happle R, Peters P, et al. Fokale dermale Hypoplasie mit apokrinen Naevi und streifenformiger Anomalie der Knochen. Arch Dermatol Res 1976;256:189–195.

7. Mehregan AH. Apocrine cystadenoma. Arch Dermatol 1964;90:274–279.

8. Kruse TV, Khan MA, Hassan MO. Multiple apocrine cystadenomas. Br J Dermatol 1979;100:675–681.

9. Smith JD, Chernosky ME. Apocrine hidrocystoma (cystadenoma). Arch Dermatol 1979;109:700–702.

10. Ahmed A, Wilson-Jones A. Apocrine cystadenoma: A report of two cases occurring on the prepuce. Br J Dermatol 1969;81:899–901.

11. Powell RF, Palmer CH, Smith EB. Apocrine cystadenoma of the penile shaft. Arch Dermatol 1977;113:1250–1251.

12. Asarch RG, Golitz LE, Sausker WF, Kreye GM. Median raphe cysts of the penis. Arch Dermatol 1979;115:1084–1086.

13. Headington JT. Mixed tumors of skin: Eccrine and apocrine types. Arch Dermatol 1961;84:989–996.

14. Hashimoto K, Eto H, Matsumoto M, Hori K. Anti-keratin monoclonal antibodies: Production, specificities and applications. J Cutan Pathol 1983;10:529–539.

15. Cramer HJ. Das schwarze Hidrocystom (Monfort). Dermatol Monatsschr 1980;166:114–118.

16. Hashimoto K, Lever WF. Appendage tumors of the skin. Springfield, Ill: Charlres C. Thomas, 1968, pp 52–54.

17. Bhawan J, Malhotra R, Frank SB. Pigmented apocrine hidrocystoma (abstr). Arch Dermatol 1980;116:1392.

18. Malhotra R, Bhawan J. The nature of pigment in pigmented apocrine hidrocystoma. J Cutan Pathol 1985;12:106–109.

19. Landry M, Winkelmann RK. An unusual tubular apocrine adenoma: Histochemical and ultrastructural study. Arch Dermatol 1972;105:869–879.

20. Umbert P, Winkelmann RK. Tubular apocrine adenoma. J Cutan Pathol 1976;3:75–87.

21. Domingo J, Helwig EB. Malignant neoplasms associated with nevus sebaceus of Jadassohn. J Am Acad Dermatol 1979;1:545–556.

22. Civatte J, Belaich S, Lauret P. Adénome tubulaire apocrine (quatre cas). Ann Dermatol Venereol 1979;106:665–669.

23. Weigand DA, Burgdorf WHC. Perianal apocrine gland adenoma. Arch Dermatol 1980;116:1051–1953.

24. Warkel RL, Helwig EB. Apocrine gland adenoma and adenocarcinoma of the axilla. Arch Dermatol 1978;114:198–203.

25. Burger RA, Marcuse PM. Fibroadenoma of the vulva. Am J Clin Pathol 1954;24:965–968.

26. Assor D, Davis JB. Multiple apocrine fibroadenomas of the anal skin. Am J Clin Pathol 1977;68:397–399.

27. Okun MR, Finn R, Blumental G. Apocrine adenoma versus apocrine carcinoma: Report of two cases. J Am Acad Dermatol 1980;2:322–326.

28. Baes H, Suurmond D. Apocrine sweat gland carcinoma: Report of a case. Br J Dermatol 1970;83:483–486.

29. Moriconi L. Adenocarcinoma delle ghiandole sudoripare. Policlinico (sez. chir.) 1931;38:634–642.

30. Stout AP, Cooley SGE. Carcinoma of sweat glands. Cancer 1951;4:521–536.

31. Ackerman LV. Surgical pathology. St. Louis: CV Mosby, 1953, p 93.

32. Elliott GB, Ramsey DW. Sweat gland carcinoma. Ann Surg 1956;144:99–106.

33. Kipkie GF, Haust MD. Carcinoma of apocrine glands: Report of a case. Arch Dermatol 1958;78:440–445.

34. Maynard JD. A case of carcinoma of an axillary apocrine gland. Br J Surg 1966;53:239–240.

35. Futrell JW, Krueger GR, Chretien PB, Ketcham AS. Multiple sweat gland carcinomas. Cancer 1971;28:686–691.

36. Tappeiner J, Wolfe K. Hidradenoma papilliferum. Eine enzymhistochemische und elektronenmikroskopische Studie. Hautarzt 1969;19:101–109.

37. Santa Cruz DJ, Prioleau PG, Smith ME. Hidradenoma papilliferum of the eyelid. Arch Dermatol 1981;117:55–56.

38. Nissim F, Czernoblisky B, Ostfeld E. Hidradenoma papilliferum of the external auditory canal. J Laryngol Otol 1981;95:843–848.

39. Meeker JH, Neubecker RD, Helwig EG. Hidradenoma papilliferum. Am J Clin Pathol 1962;37:182–195.

40. Shenoy YMV. Malignant perianal papillary hidradenoma. Arch Dermatol 1961;83:965–967.

41. Hashimoto K. Hidradenoma papilliferum: An electron microscopic study. Acta Derm Venereol (Stockh) 1973;53:22–30.

42. Helwig EB, Hackney VC. Syringoadenoma papilliferum. Arch Dermatol 1955;71:361–372.

43. Rostan SE, Waller JD. Syringocystadenoma papilliferum in an unusual location. Arch Dermatol 1976;112:835–836.

44. Premalatha S, Raghuveera Rao N, Yesudian P, Razack A, Zahra A. Segmental syringocystadenoma papilliferum in an unusual location. Int J Dermatol 1985;24:520–521.

45. Kleine-Natrop HE. Gleichzeitige Generalisation gutartiger Basaliome der beiden Typen Spiegler und Brooke. Arch Klin Exp Dermatol 1959;209:45–55.

46. Baden H. Cylindromatosis simulating neurofibromatosis. N Engl J Med 1962;267:296–297.

47. Crain RC, Helwig EB. Dermal cylindroma (dermal eccrine cylindroma). Am J Clin Pathol 1961;35:504–515.

48. Goette DK, McConnell MA, Fowler VR. Cylindroma and eccrine spiradenoma coexistent in the same lesion. Arch Dermatol 1982;118:273–274.

49. Lausecker H. Beitrag zu den Naevo-epitheliomen. Arch Dermatol Syph (Berlin) 1952;194:639–662.

50. Guggenheim W, Schnyder UW. Zur Nosologie der Spiegler-Brooke'schen Tumoren. Dermatologica 1961;122:274–278.

51. Bandmann HJ, Hamburger D, Romiti N. Bericht zur Brooke-Spieglerschen Phakomatose. Hautarzt 1965;16:450–453.

52. Welch JP, Wells RS, Kerr CB. Ancell-Spiegler cyldinromas (turban tumors) and Brooke-Fordyce trichoepitheliomas: Evidence for a single genetic entity. J Med Genet 1968;5:29–35.

53. Gottschalk HR, Graham JH, Aston EE IV. Dermal eccrine cylindroma, epithelioma adenoides cysticum, and eccrine spiradenoma. Arch Dermatol 1974;110: 473–474.

54. Headington JT, Batsakis JG, Beals TF, et al. Membranous basal cell adenoma of parotid gland, dermal cylindromas, and trichoepitheliomas. Cancer 1977; 39:2460–2469.

55. Knoth W. Epitheliomatose Phakomatose Brooke-Spiegler (Epithelioma adenoides cysticum und Zylindrome). Dermatol Monatsschr 1978;164:63–64.

56. Lever WF, Schaumburg-Lever G. Histopathology of the skin. Philadelphia: JB Lippincott, 1983, 6th ed, p 548.

57. Holubar K, Wolff K. Zur Histogenese des Cylindroms. Eine enzym-histochemische Studie. Arch Klin Exp Dermatol 1967;229:205–216.

58. Hashimoto K, Lever WF. Histogenesis of skin appendage tumors. Arch Dermatol 1969;100:356–369.

59. Munger BL, Graham JH, Helwig EB. Ultrastructure and histochemical characteristics of dermal eccrine cylindroma (turban tumor). J Invest Dermatol 1962;39:577–594.

60. Urbach F, Graham JH, Goldstein J, Munger BL. Dermal eccrine cylindroma. Arch Dermatol 1963;88:880–894.

61. Tsambaos D, Greither A, Orfanos CE. Multiple malignant Spiegler tumors with brachydactyly and racket-nails. J Cutan Pathol 1979;6:31–41.

62. Gertler W. Spieglersche Tumoren mit Übergang in metastasierendes Spinaliom. Dermatol Wochenschr 1953;128:673–674.

63. Korting GW, Hoede N, Gebhardt R. Kurzer Bericht über einen maligne entarteten Spiegler-Tumor. Dermatol Monatsschr 1960;156:141–147.

64. Luger A. Das Cylindrom der Haut und seine maligne Degeneration. Arch Dermatol Syphilis (Berlin) 1949;188:155–180.

65. Lausecker H. Beitrag zu den Naevo-epitheliomen. Arch Dermatol Syphilis (Berlin) 1952;194:639–662.

66. Lyon JB, Rouillard LM. Malignant degeneration of turban tumour of scalp. Trans St. John's Hosp Dermatol Soc 1961;46:74–77.

67. Zontschew P. Cylindroma capitis mit maligner Entartung. Zentralbl Chir 1961;86:1875–1879.

68. Bondeson L. Malignant dermal eccrine cylindroma. Acta Derm Venereol (Stockh) 1979;59:92–94.

69. Bourlond A, Clerens A, Sigard H. Cylindrome Malin. Dermatologica 1979; 158:203–207.

70. Greither A, Rehrmann A. Spiegler-Karzinome mit assoziierten Symptomen. Dermatologica 1980;160:361–370.

71. Urbanski S, From L, Abramowicz A, Joaquin A, Luk SC. Metamorphosis of dermal cylindroma: Possible relation to malignant transformation. J Am Acad Dermatol 1985;12:188–195.

72. Brownstein MH, Phelps RG, Magnin PH. Papillary adenoma of the nipple. Analysis of fifteen new cases. J Am Acad Dermatol 1985;12:707–715.

73. Dermat P, Wilson Jones E. Erosive adenomatosis of the nipple. Clin Exp Dermatol 1977;2:79–84.

74. Undeutsch W, Nikolowski J. Papillomatöses Milchgangsadenom (Pseudo-Paget der Mamille). Hautarzt 1979;30:371–375.

75. Marsch WC, Nurnberger F. Das Mamillenadenom. Z Hautkr 1979;54:1067–1072.

76. Ashikari R, Park K, Huvos AG, et al. Paget's disease of the breast. Cancer 1970;26:680–685.

77. Paone JF, Baker RR. Pathogenesis and treatment of Paget's disease of the breast. Cancer 1981;48:825–829.

78. Chrichlow RW, Czernobilsky B. Paget's disease of the male breast. Cancer 1969;24:1031–1040.

79. Hadlich J, Göring HD, Linse R. Morbus Paget beim Mann nach Östrogenbehandlung. Dermatol Monatsschr 1981;167:305–308.

80. Fligiel Z, Kaneko M. Extramammary Paget's disease of the external ear canal in association with ceruminous gland carcinoma. Cancer 1975;36:1072–1076.

81. Whorton CM, Patterson JB. Carcinoma of Moll's glands with extramammary Paget's disease of the eyelid. Cancer 1955;8:1009–1015.

82. Murrel TW Jr, McMullan FH. Extramammary Paget's disease. Arch Dermatol 1962;85:600–613.

83. Fetissoff F, Arbeille-Brassart B, Lansac J, et al. Association d'une maladie de Paget mammaire et vulvaire. Ann Dermatol Venereol 1981;109:43–50.

84. Helwig EB, Graham JH. Anogenital (extramammary) Paget's disease: A clinicopathologic study. Cancer 1963;16:387–403.

85. McKee PH, Hertogs KT. Endocervical adenocarcinoma and vulvar Paget's disease: A significant association. Br J Dermatol 1980;103:443–448.

86. Gunn RA, Gallagher HS. Vulvar Paget's disease. Cancer 1980;46:590–594.

87. Jones RE Jr, Austin C, Ackerman AB. Extramammary Paget's disease. Am J Dermatopathol 1979;1:101–132.

88. Chanda JJ. Extramammary Paget's disease: Prognosis and relationship to internal malignancy. J Am Acad Dermatol 1985;13:1009–1014.

89. Nadji M, Morales AR, Girtanner RE, Ziegels-Weissman J, Penneys NS. Paget's disease of the skin: A unifying concept of histogenesis. Cancer 1982;50:2203–2206.

90. Sasai Y, Kaji H, Natsuaki M, Nakama T. The cytoplasmic mucin in Paget cells of extramammary Paget's disease. Acta Histochem 1981;69:50–56.

91. Ishikawa E, Horiuchi R. Extramammary Paget's disease and sialic acid. Jap J Dermatol 1975;85:295–297. (Japanese).

92. Kjariniemi A-L, Ramaekers F, Lehto V-P, Virtanen I. Paget cells express cytokeratins typical of glandular epithelia. Br J Dermatol 1985;112:179–183.

93. Moll I, Moll R. Cells of extramammary Paget's disease express cytokeratins different from those of epidermal cells. J Invest Dermatol 1985;84:3–8.

94. Hashimoto K, Suzuki Y. Demonstration of eccrine type differentiation of extramammary Paget's disease by immunohistochemical methods (In preparation.)

95. Tamada S, Hirose T, Sano Y, Hinosawa K. Immunohistochemical localization of S-100 proteins in sweat gland tumors. Jap J Dermatol 1984;94:937–944.

96. Mazoujian G, Pinkus G, Haagensen DE Jr. Extramammary Paget's disease: Evidence for an apocrine origin. Am J Surg Pathol 1984;8:43–50.

97. Merot Y, Mazoujian G, Pinkus G, Momtaz-T K, Murphy GF. Extramammary Paget's disease of the perianal and perineal regions. Arch Dermatol 1985;121:750–752.

98. Haagensen DF Jr, Mazoujian G, Dilley WG, Pedersen CE, Kisler SJ, Wells SA Jr. Breast gross cystic disease fluid analysis. I. Isolation and radioimmunoassay for a major component protein. J Natl Cancer Inst 1979;62:239–247.

99. Belcher RW. Extramammary Paget's Disease. Arch Path 1972;94:59–64.

100. Ookusa Y. Histochemical studies of lectin binding pattern in human skin. I. Normal skin. Jap J Dermatol (Japanese) 1984;94:1155–1163.

101. Ookusa Y. Histochemical studies of lectin binding pattern in human skin. II. Genital Paget's disease. Jap J Dermatol 1984;94:1165–1173.

102. Medenica M, Sahihi T. Ultrastructural study of a case of extramammary Paget's disease of the vulva. Arch Dermatol 1972;105:236–243.

103. Koss LG, Brockunier A. Ultrastructural aspects of Paget's disease of the vulva. Arch Path 1969;87:592–600.

104. Caputo R, Califano A. Ultrastructural features of extramammary Paget's disease. Arch Klin Exp Derm 1970;236:212–132.

105. Demopoulos R. Fine structure of the extramammary Paget's cell. Cancer 1971;27:1202–1210.

106. Neilson D, Woodruff JD. Electron microscopy in in situ and invasive vulvar Paget's disease. Am J Obstet Gynecol 1972;113:719–732.

107. Ohyama K. Clinicopathological and electron microscopical studies on extramammary Paget's disease. II. Ultrastructure of extramammary Paget's disease. Jap J Dermatol 1981;91:1193–1206. (Japanese).

108. Ohyama K. Clinicopathological and electron microscopical studies on extramammary Paget's disease. III. Comparative study on genital and mammary Paget's disease. Jap J Dermatol 1981;91:1207–1219. (Japanese).

109. Sakamoto F, Ito M, Sato S, Sato Y. Basal cell tumor with apocrine differentiation: Apocrine epithelioma. J Am Acad Dermatol 1985;13:355–363.

110. Sato K, Leidal R, Sato F. Morphology and development of an apoeccrine sweat gland in human axillae. Am J Physiol, 1987;252:R166–180.

111. Sato K, Sato F. Sweat secretion by human axillary apoeccrine sweat gland in vitro. Am J Physiol, 1987;252:R181–187.

6

Diagnostic and Therapeutic Considerations in Patients with Skin Appendage Tumors

There are neither specific treatments nor methods of prevention for appendage tumors. An accurate diagnosis points the way to appropriate treatment. Some appendage tumors are readily identified clinically; others can be recognized with experience and careful attention, always verified by histologic findings. The purpose of this chapter is to review pertinent therapeutic considerations in patients with tumors of the skin appendages, and the diagnostic pitfalls that must be avoided so that the proper treatment will be chosen.

Treatment Considerations

The treatment of choice for almost all benign adnexal tumors of the skin is simple surgical excision. Lesions located relatively superficially may be removed by shave-type excision and electrodesiccation. A slow recurrence can be expected, however, if part of the lesion is left behind. This is true even for benign adnexal tumors such as epidermoid cysts.

In a single benign lesion such as a dilated pore of Winer or a hair follicle nevus, either complete excision for cosmetic reasons or no treatment would be the proper choice. For multiple benign tumors with no potential for malignancy, such as syringoma, steatocystoma multiplex, or trichodiscoma, no treatment would be appropriate advice; attempts to destroy these lesions can leave disfiguring scars that are worse than the original tumors. Potentially malignant varieties such as trichoepithelioma, nevus sebaceus, eccrine spiradenoma, or dermal cylindroma may be removed, when practical, by complete surgical excision. For example, it is not the practice to excise all facial lesions in multiple trichoepithelioma. However, enlarged tumors should be removed to prevent their transformation into basal cell epithelioma. Erosive, bleeding lesions (eccrine poroma) or exudative or secreting lesions (syringocystadenoma papilliferum and eccrine nevus) should be excised to prevent secondary infection. All types of eccrine gland carcinomas should be completely removed as soon as possible. Some of these tumors appear histologically rather benign but are clinically malignant because of their potential for early metastasis or deep invasion.

Sweat gland adenocarcinomas and sebaceous adenocarcinomas have an ill-defined periphery and show a marked tendency to recur following surgical excision. A wide and deep excision that includes the subcutaneous fat tissue is recommended. In complicated cases Mohs' chemosurgery or microscopically controlled excision is recommended.

Irritated portions of an adnexal tumor may show an atypical histologic picture and cytologically often appear more malignant than they actually are. This happens if one takes an infected, eroded area or previously biopsied site for histologic examination. Such artificially altered histologic findings may misguide the therapeutic decision.

Clinical Recognition

Because of their distribution, hereditary pattern, and the characteristic shape, color, and consistency of individual lesions, some types of adnexal tumors can be diagnosed clinically. These include syringoma, trichoepithelioma, steatocystoma multiplex, pilomatricoma, multiple dermal cylindroma, Fordyce's spots, and organoid nevus. Other adnexal tumors may be difficult to diagnose because they are so rare as to escape the recognition of most clinicians; examples are Muir-Torre's syndrome, Cowden's syndrome, and trichodiscoma. With some experience, the clinician can diagnose the majority of adnexal tumors if the presentation is typical; examples are eccrine poroma of the foot, trichofolliculoma with white hair, syringocystadenoma papilliferum of the scalp with an exudative and verrucous surface, eccrine spiradenoma presenting as a tender nodule, and trichilemmal cyst of the scalp.

Several tumors that usually present as subcutaneous nodules are almost impossible to diagnose clinically because they lack characteristic surface changes, such as color, texture, and configuration of the lesion, upon which dermatologists rely for identification. However, palpation of such a nodule may elicit pain (eccrine spiradenoma), or one may detect a hard consistency (pilomatricoma) or cystic fluctuation (clear cell hidradenoma). Although these signs occur in many other tumors and conditions and are not pathognomonic, they may narrow the range of clinical differential diagnosis.

Judgment on the benign versus malignant nature of an adnexal tumor should await the histologic examination. As a general rule, however, rapidity of growth, inflammatory reaction surrounding the tumor, erosion or abscess formation due to necrosis, bleeding, and pain should all be considered signs of malignancy. Some tumors are known to behave malignantly in spite of relatively benign histology; examples are eccrine carcinomas and sebaceous carcinomas of the eyelid.

Differential Diagnosis

In the differential diagnosis of the adnexal tumors, several benign and malignant lesions of the skin should be taken into consideration.

Single or multiple supernumerary nipples are often lined along the embryonal milk line and occasionally may occur elsewhere. The elevated nodular lesion is covered with an acanthotic and hyperpigmented epidermis that could be papillomatous (Fig. 6.1A). In the center are deeply invaginated excretory ducts (Fig. 6.1A) and often a group of pilosebaceous structures without hairs. Bundles of smooth muscles and groups of ectopic mammary glands are located in the underlying dermis (Fig. 6.1A, B, C).[1] The glandular component may be extensive enough to suggest a tubular apocrine adenoma or apocrine hidrocystoma (Fig. 6.2A, B, C).

An *umbilical polyp* may resemble a tubular hidradenoma. The lesion, due to the remnants of the omphaloenteric canal, exhibits gland-like structures lined with intestinal crypt epithelium that extends from the surface epidermis into the underlying dermis. The lesion is often surrounded with an inflammatory cell reaction.[2]

Mucinous syringometaplasia appears as a single hyperkeratotic growth over the plantar surface of the foot. Histologic study reveals a sinus-like dilated eccrine duct in the upper part of the tumor lined with a layer of stratified squamous epithelium. In the deeper parts the ductal epithelium shows extensive mucinous metaplasia.[3,4] The lesion exhibits marked histologic resemblance to a papillary eccrine hidradenoma.

Metastatic carcinomas to the skin should be considered in the differential diagnosis of adnexal carcinomas. Metastatic lesions of *renal cell carcinoma (hypernephroma)* to the skin consist of large cells with abundant clear cytoplasm that may resemble a clear cell eccrine carcinoma or a sebaceous adenocarcinoma (Fig. 6.3). The clear cells of hypernephroma contain glycogen granules but no lipid material.[1-3]

Metastatic adenocarcinomas to the skin[5-7] such as those originating from the thyroid (Figs. 6.4, 6.5), the breast (Fig. 6.7), or the digestive tract may exhibit glandular structures that appear similar to tubular or syringoid eccrine adenocarcinoma, apocrine adenoma, or apocrine adenocarcinomas.[2] Metastatic hepatoma to the skin (Fig. 6.6A, B) may resemble clear cell hidradenoma, sebaceous gland carcinoma, or eccrine gland carcinoma, among other entities. Metastatic lesions of breast carcinomas may exhibit epidermotropism (Fig. 6.7A, B). In the majority of metastatic lesions the dermal response is minimal, and the anaplastic tumor cells often invade the interfascicular spaces between the collagen bundles (Fig. 6.7B). Dermal lymphatics and capillary

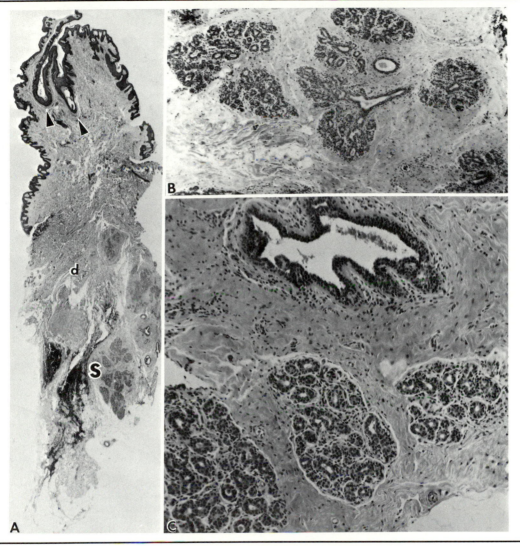

Figure 6.1

Supernumerary nipple or accessory breast from the chest wall of a young woman. An acanthotic and papillomatous surface with deeply invaginated excretion ducts (lactiferous ducts) (arrowheads) is seen in A. Secretory glands (S) and intradermal ducts (d) are situated deep at the junction of the dermis and subcutaneous adipose tissue. In B, several glandular lobules are clustered in the deep dermis. The connection of some lobules to a cystically dilated common alveolar duct is seen (see Fig. 6.2A for an enlargement). Three resting mammary glands with various alveolar cross-sections are seen in the lower half of C. In the upper half of the picture is a dilated cystic lumen, which, if alone, could be taken as an apocrine hidrocystoma (see Fig. 6.2B for an enlargement). (A, × 10; B, × 30; C, × 100.) (Courtesy of George F. Bale, M.D.)

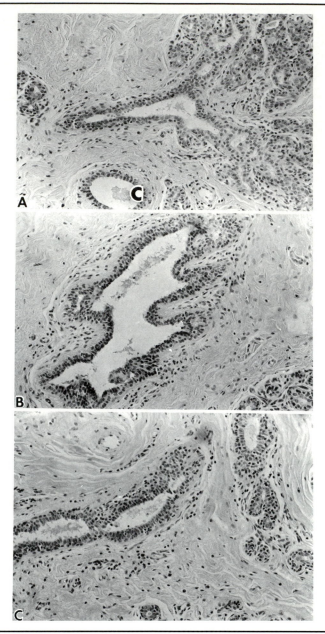

Figure 6.2
Accessory breast (same patient as in Fig. 6.1). In A, an ampulla-like dilated portion is directly connected to two lobules of resting mammary glands. This portion resembles apocrine hidrocystoma or tubular apocrine adenoma. A small cystic space (C) appears identical to the apocrine secretory portion. In B and C, cystic spaces or dilated tubular structures resemble apocrine hidrocystoma or tubular apocrine adenoma because of their tall cylindrical lining epithelium, decapitation secretion, and the products in the lumen. (A–C, × 163.)

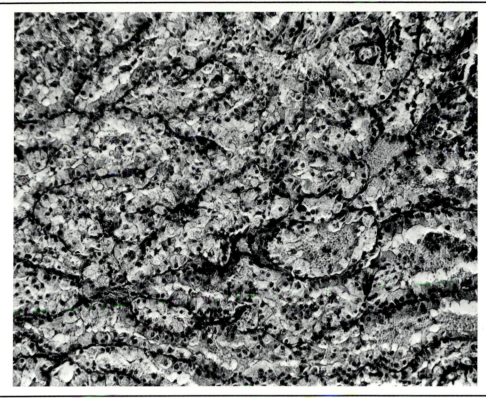

Figure 6.3
Hypernephroma metastatic to the skin. These cells are glycogen-laden clear cells and may be mistaken for eccrine gland carcinoma, clear cell schwannoma, clear cell eccrine carcinoma, or sebaceous gland adenocarcinoma among other things. (× 200.)

blood vessels may be involved. Inflammatory cell reaction is minimal. Secondary epidermal involvement and pagetoid phenomenon may be observed (Fig. 6.7A, B).[3]

REFERENCES

1. Mehregan AH. Supernumerary nipple: A histologic study. J Cutan Pathol 1981;8:96–104.
2. Mehregan AH. Pinkus' guide to dermatopathology. East Norwalk, Conn: Appleton-Century-Crofts, 1986, 4th ed.
3. King DT, Barr RJ. Syringometaplasia: Mucinous and squamous variants. J Cutan Pathol 1979;6:284–291.
4. Mehregan AH. Mucinous syringometaplasia. Arch Dermatol 1980;116:988–989.
5. Brownstein MM, Helwig EB. Spread of tumors to the skin. Arch Dermatol 1973; 107:80–86.
6. McKee PH. Cutaneous metastases. J Cutan Pathol 1985;12:239–250.
7. Mehregan AH. Metastatic carcinoma to the skin. Dermatologica 1961;123:311–325.

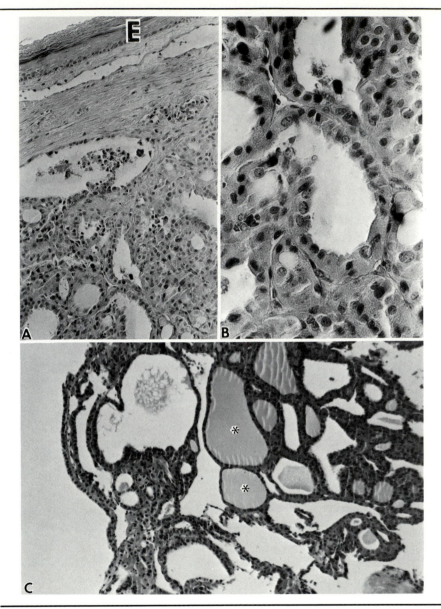

Figure 6.4
Follicular adenocarcinoma of the thyroid metastatic to the perioral skin in a 70-year-old woman. The well-differentiated adenocystic lesion strongly resembles apocrine adenoma or apocrine adenocarcinoma (A and B). In some follicles, as shown in C, colloid material is present (*) suggesting the thyroid gland origin of this tumor. E—epidermis. (A, × 163; B, × 250; C, × 130.) (Courtesy of Thomas M. Chesney, M.D.)

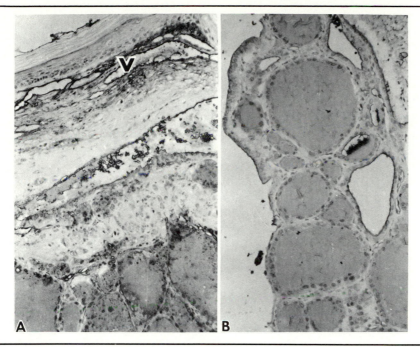

Figure 6.5
*Follicular adenocarcinoma of thyroid metastatic to the skin. Antithyroglobulin anti-
body reacts with the colloid substance and some epithelial lining cells of several follicles (A). Blood vessels (v) are nonspecifically stained with peroxidase. (B is a
control. A, × 30; B, × 50.) (Courtesy of Thomas M. Chesney, M.D.)*

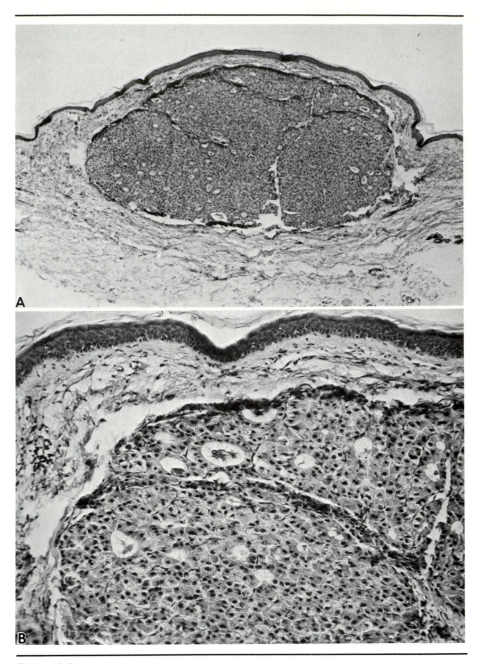

Figure 6.6
Hepatoma metastatic to the skin. (A) An intradermal nodule resembles eccrine spira-
denoma, clear cell hidradenoma, etc. (B) At higher magnification clear cells are
forming lumina or acini. This picture still resembles eccrine spiradenoma. It may
also be confused with eccrine adenocarcinoma. (A, × 20; B, × 200.)

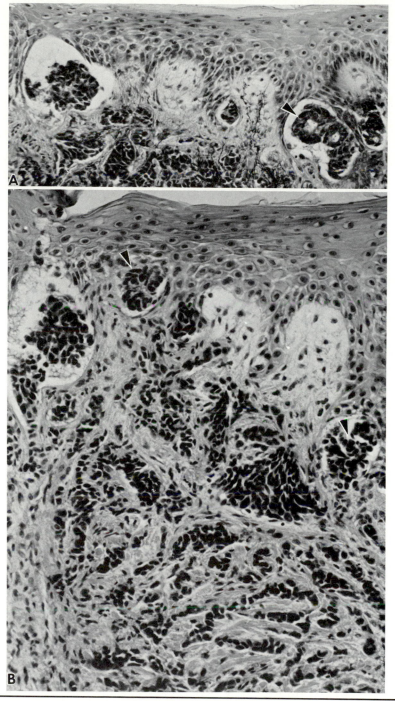

Figure 6.7
Metastatic adenocarcinoma of the breast to the skin. In A, one of the epidermotropic lesions (arrowhead) shows glandular acinus formation; this feature is also
seen in Paget's disease (cf Fig. 5.20). In B, the dermal infiltration of the tumor cells
occurs in between collagen bundles in "Indian file" fashion, whereas the epidermal
infiltration tends to form rosettes or pseudoacini (arrowhead). (A and B, × 250.)

7

Adnexal Tumors in Systemic Diseases

Some adnexal tumors are so often associated with certain systemic diseases that they constitute cutaneous markers of the systemic conditions.[1] Among these are the following entities.

Linear organoid nevi (nevus sebaceus) in a midfacial location may be associated with mental deficiency, seizures, skull changes, ocular abnormalities, porencephaly, and nonfunctioning major cerebral venous sinuses.[2–4]

Sebaceous tumors including adenoma, epithelioma, and carcinoma may be the cutaneous markers of Muir-Torre syndrome in association with multiple cancers such as adenocarcinomas of the colon, endometrium, and ovary.[5–7]

Nevus comedonicus may be associated with central nervous system disorders, including epileptiform attacks, EEG changes, and transverse myelitis as well as with skeletal abnormalities and ocular changes.[8,9]

Multiple trichilemmomas with a facial location are cutaneous markers of Cowden's disease. Other associated neoplasms are thyroid lesions, ovarian cysts, gastrointestinal polyps, and benign and malignant breast tumors.[10–12]

Multiple pilomatricomas may be associated with myotonic muscular atrophy.[13–16]

Trichoepitheliomas may be associated with lupus erythematosus.[17] The familial form may show associated vermiculate atrophoderma, milia, hypotrichosis, basal cell carcinoma, peripheral vasodilation, and cyanosis.[18]

Generalized basaloid follicular hamartoma has occurred in patients with myasthenia gravis.[19–21]

Syringomas were found in 18.5% of 200 institutionalized patients with Down's syndrome. Females were affected twice as frequently as males. Syringomas have also occurred in association with Marfan and Ehlers-Danlos syndromes.[22,23]

Eccrine poromas with multiple small lesions have been reported in a patient with hidrotic ectodermal defect.[24]

REFERENCES

1. Mehregan AH. Epithelial nevi and benign tumors of the skin and their associated systemic conditions. J Dermatol 1985;12:10–19.
2. Lovejoy FH Jr, Boyle WE Jr. Linear nevus sebaceous syndrome: Report of two cases and a review of the literature. Pediatrics 1973;52:382–387.
3. Bianchine JW. The nevus sebaceus of Jadassohn: A neurocutaneous syndrome and a potentially premalignant lesion. Amer J Dis Child 1970;120:223–228.
4. Chalub EG, Volpe JJ, Gado MH. Linear nevus sebaceus syndrome associated with porencephaly and non-functioning major cerebral venous sinuses. Neurology 1975;25:857–860.
5. Muir EG, Yates Bell AJ, Barlow KA. Multiple primary carcinomata of the colon, duodenum, and larynx associated with keratoacanthoma of the face. Br J Surg 1967;54:191–195.
6. Rulon DB, Helwig EB. Multiple sebaceous neoplasm of the skin: An association with multiple visceral carcinomas, especially of the colon. Am J Clin Pathol 1973;60:745–752.
7. Banse-Kupin L, Morales A, Barlow M. Torre's syndrome: Report of two cases and review of the literature. J Am Acad Dermatol 1984;10:803–823.
8. Engber PB. The nevus comedonicus syndrome: A case report with emphasis on associated internal manifestations. Int J Dermatol 1978;17:745–749.
9. Whyte HJ. Unilateral comedo nevus and cataract. Arch Dermatol 1968;97:533–535.
10. Brownstein MH, Mehregan AH, Bikowski JB, et al. The dermatopathology of Cowden's syndrome. Br J Dermatol 1979;100:667–673.
11. Starink TM, Hausman R. The cutaneous pathology of facial lesions in Cowden's disease. J Cutan Pathol 1984;11:331–337.
12. Salem OS, Steck WD. Cowden's disease (multiple hamartoma and neoplasia syndrome). J Am Acad Dermatol 1983;8.686–696.
13. Cantwell AR Jr, Reed WB. Myotonia atrophica and multiple calcifying epithelioma of Malherbe. Acta Derm Venereol 1965;45:387–390.
14. Harper PS. Calcifying epithelioma of Malherbe: Association with myotonic muscular dystrophy. Arch Dermatol 1972;106:41–44.
15. Chiaramonti A, Gilgor RS. Pilomatricomas associated with myotonic dystrophy. Arch Dermatol 1978;114:1363–1365.
16. Aso M, Shimao S, Takahashi K. Pilomatricomas: Association with myotonic dystrophy. Dermatologica 1981;162:197–202.
17. Winkelmann RK. Hair follicle tumors. In: Orfanos CE, and Montagna W, eds. Hair Research. Berlin: Springer Verlag, 1981.
18. Michaëlsson G, Olsson E, Westermark P. The Rombo syndrome: A familial disorder with vermiculate atrophoderma, milia, hypotrichosis, trichoepitheliomas,

basal cell carcinomas and peripheral vasodilation with cyanosis. Acta Derm Vé-néreol 1981;61:497–503.

19. Brown AC, Crounse RG, Winkelmann RK. Generalized hair follicle hamartoma. Associated with alopecia, aminoaciduria and myasthenia gravis: Report of a second case. Clin Exp Dermatol 1981;6:283–289.

20. Ridley CM, Smith N. Generalized hair follicle hamartoma associated with alopecia and myasthenia gravis: Report of a second case. Clin Exp Dermatol 1981;6:283–289.

21. Mehregan AH, Baker S. Basaloid follicular hamartoma: Report of three cases with localized and systematized unilateral lesions. J Cutan Pathol 1985;12:55–65.

22. Urban CD, Cannon JR, Cole RD. Eruptive syringomas in Down's syndrome. Arch Dermatol 1981;117:374–375.

23. Dupré A, Bonafé JL. Syringomes, mongolisme, maladie de Marfan et syndrome d'Ehlers-Danlos. Nouvelle entité posant les rapports des synringomes avec les maladies héréditaires du tissue conjonctif. Ann Derm Vénéreol 1977;104:224–230.

24. Wilkinson RD, Schopflocher P, Rozenfeld M. Hidrotic ectodermal dysplasia with diffuse eccrine poromatosis. Arch Dermatol 1977;113:472–476.

Index

Page numbers in *italic* refer to figures.